CANCER TREATMENT UPDATES 2025

A book in the Modern Medicine series

Kerry Atkinson

About this book

The painting on the front cover "Abstract Pileated woodpecker" is by Kerry Atkinson. All the text was written by the author.

Acknowledgements

I would like to acknowledge again the help that I received from Jim Severino in designing the covers for this book and for uploading it for me to Kindle Direct Publishing.

Key words: cancer, cancer treatment, oncology, chemotherapy, radiotherapy

Other books by Kerry Atkinson

Medical books

1. Graft-versus-Host Disease. Editors, S Burakoff, H J Deeg, J Ferrara, K Atkinson. Marcel Dekker Inc, New York, 1990.
2. Clinical Bone Marrow Transplantation. First edition. Editor, K Atkinson. Cambridge University Press, Cambridge UK, 1994.
3. The BMT Data Book: A Manual for Bone Marrow and Blood Stem Cell Transplantation. K. Atkinson, Cambridge University Press, Cambridge UK, 1998.
4. Clinical Bone Marrow and Blood Stem Cell Transplantation. Second Edition. Editor, K. Atkinson. Cambridge University Press, Cambridge UK, 2000.
5. Clinical Bone Marrow and Blood Stem Cell Transplantation. Third Edition. Eds, K. Atkinson, R Champlin, J Ritz, M Brenner, P Ljungman and W Fibbe. Cambridge University Press, Cambridge UK, 2004.
6. The BMT Data Book. Second edition. R Munker, HM Lazarus and K. Atkinson, Cambridge University Press, Cambridge UK, 2009.

7. The BMT Data Book: Including Cellular Therapy. Third edition. R Munker, C Hildebrandt, HM Lazarus and K. Atkinson, Cambridge University Press, Cambridge UK. 2013.
8. Hematopoietic Cell Transplants: Concepts, Controversies and Future Directions. Eds HM Lazarus, RP Gale, A Keating, A Bacigalupo, R Munker, K Atkinson, A Syed. Cambridge University Press, Cambridge, UK. 2017.
9. The Biology and Therapeutic Application of Mesenchymal Cells. Ed. K Atkinson. Wiley/Blackwell. 2017
10. Revolutionizing Tropical Medicine. Eds. K Atkinson and D Mabey. Wiley/Blackwell Publishers Inc. 2019.
11. Asthma: Targeted Biological Treatments 2020. Kindle Direct Publishing, 2020. e-book and paperback
12. Atopic Dermatitis: Targeted Biological Treatments 2020. Kindle Direct Publishing, 2020. e-book and paperback
13. Psoriasis: Targeted Biological Treatments 2020. Kindle Direct Publishing, 2020. e-book and paperback
14. Crohn's disease and ulcerative colitis: Targeted Biological Treatments 2020. Kindle Direct Publishing, 2020. e-book and paperback
15. Rheumatoid arthritis, Juvenile Idiopathic Arthritis, Ankylosing spondylitis, Psoriatic Arthritis and Gout: Targeted Biological Treatments 2020. Kindle Direct Publishing, 2020. e-book and paperback
16. Small Cell Lung Cancer: Targeted Biological Treatments 2020. Kindle Direct Publishing, 2020. e-book and paperback
17. Chronic Myeloid Leukemia: Targeted Biological Treatments 2020. Kindle Direct Publishing, 2020. e-book and paperback
18. Melanoma: Targeted Biological Treatments 2020, Kindle Direct Publishing 2020. e-book and paperback
19. Dementia - A Caregiver's Guide. Kindle Direct Publishing 2020. e-book
20. Breast Cancer: Targeted Biological Treatments 2021. Kindle Direct Publishing 2021. e-book and paperback
21. Non-melanoma Skin Cancers: Targeted Biological and Specifically Designed Therapeutic agents. 2022. Kindle Direct Publishing 2021. e-book and paperback
22. Hodgkin Lymphoma: Targeted Biological Treatments. 2022. Kindle Direct Publishing 2022. e-book and paperback

23. Chimeric Antigen Receptor (CAR) T Cells: The second Revolution in Cellular Therapy. 2022. Kindle Direct Publishing 2022. e-book and paperback
24. Acute lymphoblastic leukemia: targeted immune therapeutic agents. Kindle Direct Publishing 2023. e-book and paperback
25. Artificial Intelligence and Medicine. A book in the Modern Medicine series. Kindle Direct Publishing 2024. e-book and paperback
26. Artificial Intelligence in Medicine. Volume 2: Clinical Applications before the Availability of CHAT-GTP4. a book in the Modern Medicine series. Kindle Direct Publishing 2024. e-book and paperback
27. Check Point Inhibitors: a New Class of Drugs for Cancer Treatment. Kindle Direct Publishing 2024. e-book and paperback
28. Cancer treatment updates January 2024 – October 2024. Kindle Direct Publishing 2024. e-book and paperback

Natural history/conservation books

29. Bird facts for everyone. K Atkinson. Outskirts Press Inc., Denver, USA. 2014
30. Birds, Birds, Birds. Kindle Direct Publishing 2020. e-book and paperback
31. A Field Guide to the Wild Habitats of Sydney Australia. Kindle Direct Publishing 2021. e-book and paperback
32. Conserving New Zealand's Endangered Species. Kindle Direct Publishing 2021. e-book and paperback
33. Conserving Australia's Endangered Species. Kindle Direct Publishing 2021. e-book and paperback
34. Nature's Wonders: Britain and Ireland. Kindle Direct Publishing 2021. e-book and paperback.
35. Nature's Wonders: Spain and Bulgaria. Kindle Direct Publishing 2022. e-book and paperback.
36. Nature's Wonders: France's Camargue, the Swiss National Park and Portugal. Kindle Direct Publishing 2022. e-book and paperback.
37. Nature's Wonders: Cuba. Kindle Direct Publishing 2022. e-book and paperback.
38. Nature's Wonders: Japan in Winter Kindle Direct Publishing 2022. e-book and paperback.
39. Nature's Wonders: India. Kindle Direct Publishing 2022. e-book and paperback.

40. Nature's Wonders: Tanzania. Kindle Direct Publishing 2022. e-book and paperback.
41. The Silk Road: Uzbekistan and Kazakhstan – A Book in the Nature's Wonders Series. 2022. Kindle Direct Publishing 2022. e-book and paperback.
42. Madagascar – Land of Lemurs and Chameleons: a book in the Nature's Wonders series 2023. Kindle Direct Publishing 2022. e-book and paperback.
43. South Africa - Kalahari to the Cape - a book in the Nature's Wonders series. Kindle Direct Publishing 2022. e-book and paperback
44. Nature's Wonders – Finland - land of owls and lakes. Kindle Direct Publishing 2023. e-book and paperback
45. Nature's Wonders – Ethiopia. Kindle Direct Publishing 2023. e-book and paperback
46. Nature's Wonders – Kakadu National Park and Central Australia. Kindle Direct Publishing 2023. e-book and paperback
47. Nature's Wonders – Lord Howe Island, Australia. Kindle Direct Publishing 2023. e-book and paperback
48. Norway above the Arctic Circle in March. A book in the Nature's Wonders series. Kindle Direct Publishing 2024. e-book and paperback
49. The Inside Passage and the Pribilof Islands. A book in the Nature's Wonders series. Kindle Direct Publishing 2024. e-book and paperback
50. Orca! A book in the Nature's Wonders series. Kindle Direct Publishing 2024. e-book
51. Watching Humpback Whales from your Sofa, while sipping a Glass of Chardonnay (Australian of course) or…The Lazy Naturalist's Guide to Local Sydney Wildlife. Kindle Direct Publishing 2024. e-book and paperback
52. Magic Moments of an Amateur Naturalist. A book in the Nature's Wonder's series. Kindle Direct Publishing 2024. e-book and paperback
53. Amazing evolution Volume 1. Kindle Direct Publishing 2024. e-book and paperback
54. Nature's Wonders – the USA. Kindle Direct Publishing 2024. e-book and paperback
55. Amazing evolution Volume 2. Kindle Direct Publishing 2024. e-book and paperback

56. South Island, New Zealand. Kindle Direct Publishing 2024. e-book and paperback
57. Deserts of the World and their wildlife. Kindle Direct Publishing 2025. e-book and paperback
58. Mountain ranges of Central Asia and their wildlife. Kindle Direct Publishing 2025. e-book and paperback
59. Brisbane Birds. A book in the Nature's Wonders series. Kindle Direct Publishing 2025. e-book and paperback
60. Amazing evolution Volume 3. Snow leopards, Ivory-billed woodpeckers, Spoon-billed sandpipers and more. Kindle Direct Publishing 2025. e-book and paperback
61. Lake Baikal and its wildlife. A book in the Nature's Wonders series. Kindle Direct Publishing 2025. e-book and paperback
62. Little known seas of the World and their wildlife. Kindle Direct Publishing 2025. e-book and paperback
63. Amazing Evolution Volume 4: the Wily Hedge sparrow, Strange-shaped beaks, iridescent feathers and more. A book in the Nature's Wonders series. Kindle Direct Publishing 2025. e-book and paperback
64. Driving the Pamir Highway in Tajikistan 2025. A book in the Nature's Wonders series. Kindle Direct Publishing 2025. e-book and paperback
65. The Aleutian Islands and their Wildlife – the Pacific Rim of Fire. A book in the Nature's Wonders series. Kindle Direct Publishing 2025. e-book and paperback
66. Amazing Evolution Volume 5.: Pangolins, Emus that swim, Axolotls that re-grow severed limbs and more. Kindle Direct Publishing 2025. e-book and paperback

Other books

67. Paintings by Kerry Atkinson 2019 – 2021. Kindle Direct Publishing 2021. e-book and paperback.
68. Ferrari Road Cars. Kindle Direct Publishing 2022. e-book and paperback.
69. Paintings by Kerry Atkinson. 2022. Kindle Direct Publishing 2022. e-book and paperback.

70. Samuel Beckett and Bob Dylan – living in a Shakespearean era. Kindle Direct Publishing 2022. e-book and paperback.
71. Paintings and sculptures by Kerry Atkinson 2023. Kindle Direct Publishing 2023. e-book and paperback.
72. Ten influential European paintings. Kindle Direct Publishing 2023. e-book and paperback
73. The Pillars of Rock 'N Roll. Kindle Direct Publishing 2024. e-book and paperback
74. Early 20th Century Western paintings - a smorgasbord of color and radical shapes. Kindle Direct Publishing 2024. e-book
75. Insects and other wildlife included in Dutch flower paintings from the Dutch golden age. Kindle Direct Publishing 2024. e-book and paperback
76. Paintings and sculptures by Kerry Atkinson 2024. Kindle Direct Publishing 2024. e-book and paperback
77. Ferrari Road Cars. Kindle Direct Publishing 2022. e-book and paperback
78. Samuel Beckett and Bob Dylan – living in a Shakespearean era. Kindle Direct Publishing 2022. e-book and paperback
79. The Pillars of Rock 'N Roll. Kindle Direct Publishing 2024. e-book and pap
80. Paintings and sculptures by Kerry Atkinson 2024. Kindle Direct Publishing 2025. e-book and paperback
81. Cadillacs with Rocket-like Tailfins. Kindle Direct Publishing 2025. e-book and paperback
82. Boy Racer. Kindle Direct Publishing 2025. e-book and paperback
83. Paintings and sculptures by Kerry Atkinson 2025. Kindle Direct Publishing 2025.

TABLE OF CONTENTS

1. Author's preface, page 10

Diseases

2. Non-small cell lung cancer, page 10
3. Small cell lung cancer, page 19
4. Breast cancer, page 20
5. Colo-rectal cancer, page 45
6. Anal cancer, page 60
7. Prostate cancer, page 61
8. Bladder/urothelial cancer, page 68
9. Renal cancer, page 71
10. Head and neck cancer, page 73
11. Gastric carcinoma and esophogastric carcinoma, page 79
12. Pancreatic cancer, page 86
13. Melanoma, page 86
14. Non-melanoma skin cancers, page 88
15. Endometrial cancer, page 91
16. Carcinoma of the cervix, page 92
17. Carcinoma of the thyroid, page 94
18. Biliary tract neoplasms, page 95
19. Hepatocellular carcinoma, page 96
20. Neuroendocrine cancers, page 100
21. Cancer of unknown primary site, page 102
22. Non-Hodgkin lymphoma, page 108
23. Hodgkin lymphoma, page 118
24. Chronic lymphocytic leukemia, page 121
25. Acute lymphoblastic leukemia, page 125
26. Acute promyelocytic leukemia, page 130
27. Myeloma, page 131

28. Myelofibrosis, page 135

Other developments in cancer medicine

29. RSV Vaccination in Stem-Cell Transplant Recipients, page 136

30. Anticoagulation in Patients with Cancer-Associated Pulmonary Embolism: How Long Is Long Enough, page 137

31. Apixaban for Extended Treatment of Provoked Venous Thromboembolism, page 137

32. Anticoagulation and Intracranial Hemorrhage in Patients with Brain Metastases, page 139

33. Medical Imaging and Risk for Blood Cancers in Children and Adolescents, page 140

34. A Pathway to Immunotherapeutic Targeting of Multiple Cancer Types, page 141

35. How to Prevent Chemotherapy-Induced Peripheral Neuropathy, page 142

36. GLP-1 Receptor Agonist Use and Cancer Risk, page 143

37. Overall Cancer Risk after HPV Vaccination, page 144

38. Covid-19 mRNA Vaccines Aid Immune Checkpoint Inhibitor Cancer Therapy, page 145

39. Caring for Long-Term Survivors of Childhood Cancer, page 145

40. Conclusions, page 146

41. References, page 146

42. Abbreviations used, page 155

1. Author's Preface

Oncology continues to be one of the main beneficiaries, if not the main beneficiary, of the research revolution in biology and biomedical science that has occurred over the past 5 decades. As well as surgery, radiotherapy, and chemotherapy, another type of cancer treatment has been introduced recently – immunotherapy in the form of monoclonal antibodies – now applied to most types of cancer as checkpoint inhibitors to inhibit the suppression by cancers of the human immune system, unleashing it to play its role in the anti-cancer attack. For the first time cure is on the horizon for tumors previously thought to be uniformly fatal: advanced melanoma and non-small cell lung cancer are examples. The tsunami of new drugs continues unabated and a second type of cell therapy has entered mainstream medicine - chimeric antigen reactive T cells. Because of all this new knowledge I think it unlikely that there will be a role for general medical oncologists on the future: medical oncologists will likely follow the example of the previous specialization of general physicians, probably specializing in one of the big four carcinomas while keeping in sufficient touch with the literature to be able to pay a useful part in the management of less common cancers

1. NON-SMALL CELL LUNG CANCER

Screening for lung cancer[100]

A calculator, which is easy to use online, can help inform conversations with patients: an individualized cancer risk estimate might be exactly what someone sitting on the fence needs to feel more comfortable about choosing screening.

Eligibility for lung cancer screening in some countries is based solely on age and smoking history, but multiple studies have shown that a more personalized risk assessment, incorporating other known risk factors, might better identify patients who could benefit from screening.

Researchers in Germany compared the performance of the Nelson criteria, which are similar to the U.S. criteria, against a previously validated risk calculator (PLCOm2012) that takes into account not only age and smoking history but also race, education, personal and family history of cancer, body-mass index, and chronic obstructive pulmonary disease. The study involved 5000 individuals who met the Nelson criteria or were at elevated risk for lung cancer according to the risk calculator (6-year risk, ≥1.6%). All participants underwent initial low-dose CT followed by repeat screening at 1 year

Slightly more individuals were identified by the risk calculator than by the Nelson criteria (80% vs. 75%). Altogether, 111 cancers were detected; the number detected was higher in the group identified by the calculator than by the Nelson criteria (108 vs. 85 cancers).

Overall Survival with Neoadjuvant Nivolumab plus Chemotherapy in Lung Cancer[55]

Three cycles of neoadjuvant nivolumab plus chemotherapy significantly improved overall survival among patients with resectable NSCLC as compared with chemotherapy alone.

In this open-label, phase 3 trial, patients with stage IB to IIIA resectable NSCLC were randomly assigned to receive nivolumab plus chemotherapy or chemotherapy alone for three cycles, followed by surgery. The primary end points were event-free survival and pathological complete response. The investigators reorted the results of the planned analysis of overall survival.

A total of 358 patients were concurrently assigned to receive nivolumab plus chemotherapy (179 patients) or chemotherapy alone (179 patients). The final analysis of overall survival significantly favored neoadjuvant nivolumab plus chemotherapy over chemotherapy (hazard ratio for death, 0.72; 95% confidence interval [CI], 0.523 to 0.998; P=0.048). At a median follow-up of 68.4 months, the 5-year overall survival was 65.4% with nivolumab plus chemotherapy and 55.0% with chemotherapy alone, with consistency across most subgroups. In exploratory analyses, the 5-year overall survival in the nivolumab-plus-chemotherapy group was 95.3% (95% CI, 82.7 to 98.8) among the patients with a pathological complete response and 55.7% (95% CI, 46.9 to 63.7) among those without such a response; Survival was 75.0% among the patients with presurgery clearance of circulating tumor DNA (ctDNA) and 52.6% among those without such clearance.

No new safety signals were observed.

No data were presented regarding the possible increased risk from nivolumab on the subsequent lung surgery.

Smoking Cessation Programs for Cancer Patients[98]

On average, patients who stopped smoking lived longer, especially those who stopped sooner after their cancer was diagnosed.

Smoking raises risk for all-cause and cancer-specific deaths in patients with cancer - even among patients with cancers for which smoking is not a major risk factor. However, not all smokers with cancer receive formal tobacco-cessation management. In a prospective cohort study, researchers looked at survival outcomes in 4,526 smokers who received diagnoses of any type of cancer and who subsequently were enrolled in a tobacco intervention program at MD Anderson Cancer Center. The program consisted of multiple counselling visits and personalized medication treatment.

Among patients who enrolled in the program within 6 months of their cancer diagnoses, the group who reported having stopped smoking at 3 months had significantly longer survival than did non-quitters (71% vs. 61% for 5-year survival; 58% vs. 52% for 10-year survival). Patients who enrolled between 6 months and 5 years after their cancer was diagnosed and who subsequently quit also had longer survival, as did patients who quit by 6 or 9 months (rather than just 3 months) after enrolment. However, those who enrolled and quit smoking longer than 5 years after their cancer was diagnosed did not have a survival benefit over those who continued to smoke.

Sevabertinib in Advanced *HER2*-Mutant Non–Small-Cell Lung Cancer[112]

HER2 gene mutations occur in 2 to 4% of patients with non–small-cell lung cancer (NSCLC). Sevabertinib is an oral, reversible tyrosine kinase inhibitor that has shown anti-HER2 activity in preclinical models.

The investigators conducted an open-label, multicenter, multicohort, phase 1–2 study to evaluate sevabertinib at a twice-daily dose of 20 mg in patients with locally advanced or metastatic HER2-mutant NSCLC. Three cohorts were defined according to previous therapy: cohort D comprised previously treated patients who had not received HER2-targeted therapy; cohort E, patients who had previously received HER2-directed antibody–drug conjugates; and cohort F, patients who had not previously received treatment. The primary end point was an objective response, as assessed by blinded independent central review. Secondary end points were duration of response and progression-free survival.

A total of 209 patients received sevabertinib (as of June 27, 2025, the data-cutoff date); the median duration of follow-up was 13.8 months in cohort D, 11.7 months in cohort E, and 9.9 months in cohort F. Among 81 patients in cohort D, an objective response was observed in 64% (95% confidence interval [CI], 53 to 75); the median duration of response was 9.2 months (95% CI, 6.3 to 13.5), and the median progression-free survival was 8.3 months (95% CI, 6.9 to 12.3). Among 55 patients in cohort E, an objective response was observed in 38% (95% CI, 25 to 52); the median duration of response was 8.5 months, and the median progression-free survival was 5.5 months. Among 73 patients in cohort F, an objective response was observed in 71% (95% CI, 59 to 81), and the median duration of response was 11.0 months; data on progression-free survival were immature. Grade 3 or higher drug-related adverse events occurred in 31% of the patients. The most common adverse event was diarrhea (in 84 to 91%), with diarrhea of grade 3 or higher occurring in 5 to 23%. Treatment was discontinued by 3% of the patients owing to drug-related adverse event. Sevabertinib showed antitumor activity in patients with locally advanced or metastatic HER2-mutant NSCLC. Diarrhea was the most common adverse event.

Updated American Society of Clinical Oncology (ASCO) Guidelines for Treating Stage IV Non–Small Cell Lung Cancer[57]

Non–small cell lung cancer (NSCLC) comprises a multitude of biomarker-driven diseases. The authors highlighted two ASCO guidelines on stage IV NSCLC on the need for biomarker analysis in treatment decisions and showed the array of treatment options. ASCO publishes these "living" guidelines on a regular schedule due to the pace of research in the field. Clinicians should no longer think of "stage IV NSCLC" as a single category. The very first action for treating clinicians is to obtain full molecular and PD-L1 testing on the timor. While some new treatment combinations look interesting, none changes first-line standards today. What matters most is making sure every patient has access to comprehensive testing up front.

Start with testing for tumor drivers. At diagnosis, order a tissue or blood-based multigene panel. At minimum, look for mutations in EGFR, HER2, BRAF, KRAS;

rearrangements in ALK, ROS1, RET, NTRK, NRG1; and MET exon 14 skipping. Use immunohistochemistry to check for PD-L1 and HER2.

If a driver is present, target therapy to the driver. If testing identifies a driver alteration, targeted therapy is critical and often the preferred first-line treatment, depending on the alteration. At progression, retesting can uncover new resistance mechanisms to the target.

If no driver is present, use PD-L1. Here, immunotherapy — alone or combined with chemotherapy — remains the foundation of care.

Integrate palliative care early. Alongside any treatment path, early integration of palliative care improves quality of life.

The guidelines note new but not practice-changing findings:

The RAMOSE trial added ramucirumab to osimertinib in EGFR-mutated disease, modestly improving progression-free survival, but methodological issues preclude changes in guidance for first-line EGFR treatment.

In a phase 2 trial, zenocutuzumab showed promise in NRG1 fusion, a rare event in solid tumors, with a 29% response rate, supporting its use in this population.

Trials of dual checkpoint blockade or ivonescimab, a novel bispecific VEGF and PD-1 antibody, showed mixed efficacy and higher toxicity, leaving standard regimens unchanged.

Overall Survival with Amivantamab–Lazertinib in EGFR-Mutated Advanced NSC[120]

Previous results from this phase 3 trial showed that progression-free survival among participants with previously untreated EGFR (epidermal growth factor receptor)–mutated advanced non–small-cell lung cancer (NSCLC) was significantly improved with amivantamab–lazertinib as compared with osimertinib. Results of the protocol-specified final overall survival analysis in this trial have not been reported.

The investigators randomly assigned, in a 2:2:1 ratio, participants with previously untreated EGFR-mutated (exon 19 deletion or L858R substitution), locally advanced or metastatic NSCLC to receive amivantamab–lazertinib, osimertinib, or lazertinib. Overall survival (assessed in an analysis of the time from randomization to death from any cause) in the amivantamab–lazertinib group as compared with the osimertinib group was a key secondary end point. Additional end points included safety.

A total of 429 participants each were assigned to receive amivantamab–lazertinib or osimertinib. Over a median follow-up of 37.8 months, amivantamab–lazertinib led to significantly longer overall survival than osimertinib (hazard ratio for death, 0.75; 95% confidence interval, 0.61 to 0.92; P=0.005); 3-year overall survival was 60% and 51%, respectively. At the clinical cutoff date, 38% of participants in the amivantamab–lazertinib group and 28% in the osimertinib group were still receiving the assigned treatment. Adverse events of grade 3 or higher were more common with amivantamab–lazertinib (in 80% of participants) than with osimertinib (in 52%), particularly skin-related events, venous thromboembolism, and infusion-related events; these findings were consistent with the established safety profile of each treatment. No new safety signals were observed with additional follow-up.

Amivantinab–lazertinib led to significantly longer overall survival among participants with previously untreated EGFR-mutated advanced NSCLC than osimertinib but was associated with an increased risk of adverse events of grade 3 or higher.

Sacituzumab Tirumotecan in EGFR-TKI–Resistant, EGFR-Mutated Advanced NSCL[125]

In patients with EGFR-mutated advanced or metastatic NSCLC that had progressed after previous EGFR-TKI therapy, progression-free survival and overall survival outcomes were significantly better with sac-TMT than with platinum-based chemotherapy

Sacituzumab tirumotecan (sac-TMT) is an antibody–drug conjugate targeting trophoblast cell-surface antigen 2 that has shown significant survival benefits in patients with EGFR-mutated non–small-cell lung cancer (NSCLC) that has progressed after epidermal growth factor receptor (EGFR) tyrosine kinase inhibitor (TKI) therapy and platinum-based chemotherapy.

In this phase 3 trial, the investigators enrolled patients with EGFR-mutated locally advanced or metastatic nonsquamous NSCLC that had progressed after EGFR-TKI therapy. The patients were randomly assigned, in a 1:1 ratio, to receive sac-TMT monotherapy or pemetrexed plus platinum-based chemotherapy. The primary end point was progression-free survival as assessed by blinded independent review. Overall survival was a hierarchically tested key secondary end point. In the interim analysis of progression-free survival as assessed by blinded independent review, sac-TMT monotherapy met the prespecified criterion for significance (two-sided P<0.0001); the investigators reported here the prespecified final analysis of progression-free survival and the preplanned interim analysis of overall survival.

Overall, 376 patients underwent randomization, with 188 assigned to each group. After a median follow-up of 18.9 months, the median progression-free survival was 8.3 months in the sac-TMT group and 4.3 months in the chemotherapy group (hazard ratio for disease progression or death, 0.49; 95% confidence interval [CI], 0.39 to 0.62). Overall survival was significantly longer with sac-TMT than with chemotherapy (hazard ratio for death, 0.60; 95% CI, 0.44 to 0.82; two-sided P=0.001); 18-month overall survival was 65.8% and 48.0%, respectively. Treatment-related adverse events of grade 3 or higher occurred in 58.0% of patients receiving sac-TMT and in 53.8% of those receiving chemotherapy, with the most common being a decreased neutrophil count (39.9% vs. 33.0%); treatment-related serious adverse events occurred in 9.0% and 17.6%, respectively.

A New First-Line Standard for EGFR-Mutated NSCLC?[115]

First-line treatment of patients with EGFR-mutated NSCLC with osimertinib and platinum-pemetrexed chemotherapy leads to significantly longer overall survival than osimertinib alone.

Among patients with non–small-cell lung cancer (NSCLC) and sensitizing mutations in the epidermal growth factor receptor (EGFR) gene, the primacy of first-line osimertinib monotherapy has been challenged by two combination regimens. The MARIPOSA trial showed progression-free survival (PFS) and overall-survival (OS) benefits of amivantamab–lazertinib over osimertinib alone. The phase 3, open-label FLAURA2 trial previously showed a PFS benefit of platinum-pemetrexed chemotherapy with osimertinib over osimertinib alone. The current update reported OS results, a key secondary end point. Investigators randomized 557 patients with locally advanced or metastatic NSCLC and sensitizing EGFR mutations to first-line treatment with osimertinib plus platinum-pemetrexed chemotherapy (four induction cycles of platinum doublet, followed by maintenance with a median 11 cycles of pemetrexed, with daily osimertinib throughout) or to osimertinib alone.

Median OS was significantly longer with combination therapy than with osimertinib alone: 48 months versus 38 months. OS benefit occurred among patients with and without brain metastases and with either L858R or exon 19 deletion.

The median duration of osimertinib exposure was 31 months in the combination-therapy group and 21 months in the monotherapy group.

The combination-therapy group had a higher rate of grade 3 or higher adverse events (70% vs. 34%), most commonly anemia, neutropenia, and decreased platelet count. Onset of adverse events with combination therapy was most frequent during induction and decreased during maintenance

Two large randomized studies now show superior overall survival with combination treatment over osimertinib monotherapy in the first line treatment of EGFR-mutated advanced NSCLC — although at the cost of increased toxicity.

Zongertinib in Previously Treated HER2-Mutant NSCLC[131]

Zongertinib showed clinical benefit with mainly low-grade adverse events in patients with previously treated HER2-mutant NSCLC.

Innovative oral targeted therapies are warranted for patients with human epidermal growth factor receptor 2 (*HER2*)–mutant non–small-cell lung cancer (NSCLC). Zongertinib is an oral, irreversible, HER2-selective tyrosine kinase inhibitor that has been shown to have efficacy in persons with advanced or metastatic solid tumors with HER2 alterations in a phase 1 study.

The investigators evaluated zongertinib in a multicohort, phase 1a–1b trial involving patients with advanced or metastatic *HER2*-mutant NSCLC. Here they reported the primary analysis of zongertinib in previously treated patients: those with tumors harboring a mutation in the tyrosine kinase domain (cohort 1), those with tumors harboring a mutation in the tyrosine kinase domain previously treated with a HER2-directed antibody–drug conjugate (cohort 5), and those with tumors harboring a non–tyrosine kinase domain mutation (cohort 3).

In cohort 1, patients were initially randomly assigned to receive zongertinib at a dose of 120 mg or 240 mg once daily. Patients in cohorts 5 and 3 initially received 240 mg daily. After an interim analysis of data from cohort 1, subsequently recruited patients across all cohorts received zongertinib at a dose of 120 mg. The primary end point was an objective response assessed by blinded independent central review (cohorts 1 and 5) or by investigator review (cohort 3). Secondary end points included the duration of response and progression-free survival.

In cohort 1, a total of 75 patients received zongertinib at a dose of 120 mg. At the data cutoff (November 29, 2024), 71% of these patients (95% confidence interval [CI], 60 to 80; $P<0.001$ against a ≤30% benchmark) had a confirmed objective response; the median duration of response was 14.1 months (95% CI, 6.9 to not evaluable), and the median progression-free survival was 12.4 months (95% CI, 8.2 to not evaluable). Grade 3 or higher drug-related adverse events occurred in 13 patients (17%). In cohort 5 (31 patients), 48% of the patients (95% CI, 32 to 65) had a confirmed objective response. Grade 3 or higher drug-related adverse events occurred in 1 patient (3%). In cohort 3 (20 patients), 30% of the patients (95% CI, 15 to 52) had a confirmed objective response. Grade 3 or higher drug-related adverse events occurred in 5 patients (25%). Across all three cohorts, no cases of drug-related interstitial lung disease occurred.

Overall Survival with Neoadjuvant Nivolumab plus Chemotherapy in Lung Cancer[133]

Three cycles of neoadjuvant nivolumab plus chemotherapy significantly improved overall survival among patients with resectable NSCLC as compared with chemotherapy alone.

Neoadjuvant nivolumab plus chemotherapy significantly improved pathological complete response and event-free survival in patients with resectable non–small-cell lung cancer (NSCLC) in a phase 3 trial. Data are needed on overall survival.

In this open-label, phase 3 trial, patients with stage IB to IIIA resectable NSCLC were randomly assigned to receive nivolumab plus chemotherapy or chemotherapy alone for three cycles, followed by surgery. The primary end points were event-free survival and pathological complete response. The investigators reported the results of the planned analysis of overall survival.

A total of 358 patients were concurrently assigned to receive nivolumab plus chemotherapy (179 patients) or chemotherapy alone (179 patients). The final analysis of overall survival significantly favored neoadjuvant nivolumab plus chemotherapy over chemotherapy (hazard ratio for death, 0.72; 95% confidence interval [CI], 0.523 to 0.998; P=0.048). At a median follow-up of 68.4 months, the 5-year overall survival was 65.4% with nivolumab plus chemotherapy and 55.0% with chemotherapy alone, with consistency across most subgroups. In exploratory analyses, the 5-year overall survival in the nivolumab-plus-chemotherapy group was 95.3% (95% CI, 82.7 to 98.8) among the patients with a pathological complete response and 55.7% (95% CI, 46.9 to 63.7) among those without such a response; survival was 75.0% among the patients with presurgery clearance of circulating tumor DNA (ctDNA) and 52.6% among those without such clearance. No new safety signals were observed.

Three cycles of neoadjuvant nivolumab plus chemotherapy significantly improved overall survival among patients with resectable NSCLC as compared with chemotherapy alone.

2. SMALL CELL LUNG CANCER

A New Second-Line Treatment for Small-Cell Lung Cancer?[74]

Immunotherapy with tarlatamab resulted in better overall survival than standard second-line chemotherapies.

While initial response rates to standard first-line treatment of extensive-stage small-cell lung cancer are high, disease almost invariably recurs. Current second-line options include chemotherapies such as topotecan or lurbinectedin in the United States and amrubicin in Japan. Tarlatamab, a novel class of therapy, is a bispecific T-cell engager targeting DLL3 on tumor cells and CD3 on T cells, enabling T-cell–mediated immunologic destruction of tumor cells. DeLLphi-304, an international, randomized, phase 3 trial, compared tarlatamab with chemotherapy (topotecan, lurbinectedin, or amrubicin) in approximately 500 adults with extensive small-cell lung cancer who progressed on or after standard first-line treatment.

The results of an interim analysis were as follows:

- Tarlatamab resulted in significantly longer overall survival compared to standard second-line chemotherapies (median, 13.6 vs. 8.3 months).
- Progression-free survival and cancer-related symptoms such as dyspnea and cough were significantly better with tarlatamab.

Cytokine release syndrome (CRS) was the most common adverse event seen with tarlatamab; most events occurred with the first two doses and were low grade.

Immune effector cell–associated neurotoxicity syndrome (ICANS) was rare.

This study establishes tarlatamab as the new standard second-line treatment for extensive-stage small-cell lung cancer. There are special considerations with tarlatamab, including the need for inpatient monitoring of CRS and ICANS for the first few doses. However, subsequent treatments can usually be safely moved to the outpatient setting.

3. BREAST CANCER

Response–Guided Axillary Treatment of Node-Positive Breast Cancer: The MARI Protocol[51]

In patients with limited nodal disease, the post-MARI risk for axillary recurrence was very low

(MARI: marking the axillary lymph node with a radioactive seed)

The quest to de-escalate therapy for breast cancer has prompted tailored axillary lymph node dissection, modified radiation therapy (RT) protocols, and fewer mastectomies; but do these less-intense treatments raise recurrence risk, thereby compromising survival? Investigators in the Netherlands pursued the "marking the axillary lymph node with a radioactive seed" (MARI) protocol in patients with operable breast cancer and node-positive disease. Those who attained a pathologic complete response (pCR) in the MARI node following primary systemic treatment (PST) received no further axillary treatment, while those with residual disease received RT including the axilla. Patients undergoing breast-conserving surgery (BCS) received RT to the breast. Those with residual nodal disease at surgery received RT to the breast or chest wall as well as the axilla. The primary outcome was axillary recurrence rate; secondary outcomes included invasive disease-free survival (iDFS) and overall survival (OS).

350 patients (median age 49 years) were enrolled from 2014–2021 with a median follow-up of 49 months. Among 135 patients, pCR of the MARI node was confirmed, whereas 215 had residual disease. Most patients (65%) underwent BCS. In patients with pCR in the MARI node, the axillary recurrence rate was 0.7%, 5-year iDFS was 93%, and OS was 98%, while among patients with residual disease in the MARI node, axillary recurrence occurred in 2.3%, with iDFS of 82% and OS of 93%.

These data suggest that patients who have low nodal burden before and who attain pCR in the MARI node have a very low risk for local recurrence and excellent overall outcomes.

Sequential Cytotoxic Payloads Against Metastatic Breast Cancer[52]

In a retrospective observational study, treatment with sacituzumab govitecan after T-DXd was associated with shorter progression-free survival.

The use of antibody-drug conjugates (ADCs, wherein an antitumor antibody is linked to a cytotoxic payload) has improved outcomes across many tumor types. For the three ADCs thus far approved in the setting of breast cancer, the payload is a topoisomerase 1 inhibitor: trastuzumab deruxtecan (T-DXd), sacituzumab govitecan (SG), or datopotamab deruxtecan. T-DXd is used for HER2-positive metastatic breast cancer as well as HER2-low and HER2-ultralow disease (including endocrine-refractory disease).

The investigators conducted a retrospective observational study of a database spanning 280 USA clinics. Patients who received T-DXd and at least one additional non–T-DXd therapy between 2019 and 2023 were included, and tumors were defined as HER2-positive, HER2-low, or HER2-0 based on the most recent biopsy. The primary endpoint was PFS (PFS).

A total of 793 patients were identified who had received another line of systemic therapy after discontinuing T-DXd, most often because of disease progression. Tumor types were HER2-positive (54%), ER-positive/HER2-negative (37%), and triple negative (~10%). Across all patients and subtypes, after adjustment for prior lines of treatment, treatment with SG after T-DXd was associated with shorter PFS relative to the other regimens (3.4 months vs. 5.0 months).

Other smaller studies have indicated a similarly poor PFS when two topisomerase 1 inhibitor ADCs are given in sequence. These findings suggest a mechanism of resistance due to similar payloads. The selection of therapy following disease progression on T-DXd should ensure that a specific cytotoxic payload is used. Alternatively, other treatment options such as chemotherapy or different targeted therapies may be appropriate (whether HER2-directed or endocrine-based)

Breast Cancer Risk in Women Receiving No or Delayed Treatment for DCIS[53]

The estimated 8-year incidence of ipsilateral invasive breast cancer was relatively low at 11%.

Standard treatment for ductal carcinoma in situ (DCIS) includes surgery, often with radiation and endocrine therapy, but its favorable prognosis has generated concern about overtreatment. In a recent randomized trial, active monitoring of low-risk DCIS was not associated with increased risk of invasive breast cancer compared with standard care; longer-term follow-up is pending. Meanwhile, observational studies offer further evidence to inform clinical decision making. In the current one, researchers assessed the risk of subsequent ipsilateral invasive Chapter in 1800 USA women with biopsy-confirmed DCIS who received no surgery or radiation within six months of diagnosis. 38% of women eventually had surgery and 25% received endocrine therapy.

During a median follow-up of 5 years, 7% developed invasive breast cancer, and breast cancer mortality was 1.6%. The estimated 8-year cumulative incidence of invasive breast cancer was 11%, ranging from 9% in women with low-risk DCIS (defined as low-grade histology, hormone receptor–positive, and age ≥40) to 14% in those with high-risk DCIS.

The reasons for delayed or absent treatment in these patients are unknown, and this was not a study of active surveillance. Nonetheless, the risk for invasive breast cancer after a DCIS diagnosis was low, as noted by the authors; the range is similar to the risk associated with benign atypia, which is often managed with surveillance. The management of low-risk DCIS will continue to evolve as clinicians and patients weigh overtreatment against the risk of invasive breast cancer. Several ongoing randomized trials will help clarify the best strategies for low-risk DCIS. For now, patients can be reassured that short-term delays in treatment are unlikely to increase their risk for invasive breast cancer.

Elinzanetant for Vasomotor Symptoms from Endocrine Therapy for Breast Cancer[54]

Elinzanetant led to a significantly lower frequency of vasomotor symptoms associated with endocrine therapy than placebo

Women receiving endocrine therapy for hormone receptor (HR)–positive breast cancer, or those at high risk for breast cancer, commonly have vasomotor symptoms (hot flashes). Elinzanetant, a neurokinin-targeted therapy.

The investigators performed a phase 3 trial involving women 18 to 70 years of age with moderate-to-severe vasomotor symptoms associated with endocrine therapy for HR-positive breast cancer or its prevention. Women were randomly assigned in a 2:1 ratio to receive once-daily elinzanetant at a dose of 120 mg for 52 weeks or once-daily placebo for 12 weeks followed by once-daily elinzanetant at a dose of 120 mg for 40 weeks. The primary end points were the change in the mean daily frequency of moderate-to-severe vasomotor symptoms from baseline to week 4 and to week 12.

A total of 316 participants were assigned to the elinzanetant group and 158 to the placebo–elinzanetant group. At baseline, the mean daily frequency of moderate-to-severe vasomotor symptoms was 11.4 episodes (95% confidence interval [CI], 10.7 to 12.2) in the elinzanetant group and 11.5 episodes (95% CI, 10.5 to 12.5) in the placebo–elinzanetant group. At week 4, the mean change from baseline in the mean daily frequency of moderate-to-severe vasomotor symptoms was −6.5 episodes (95% CI, −7.2 to −5.8) among those who were receiving elinzanetant and −3.0 episodes (95% CI, −3.9 to −2.2) among those who were receiving placebo (P<0.001). At week 12, the mean change was −7.8 episodes (95% CI, −8.5 to −7.1) among those receiving elinzanetant and −4.2 episodes (95% CI, −5.2 to −3.2) among those receiving placebo (P<0.001). During weeks 1 through 12, a total of 220 participants (69.8%) receiving elinzanetant and 98 (62.0%) receiving placebo reported at least one adverse event that occurred while receiving elinzanetant or placebo, with the most common being headache, fatigue, and somnolence. Serious adverse events occurred during weeks 1 through 12 in 8 participants (2.5%) receiving elinzanetant and 1 participant (0.6%) receiving placebo.

How to Improve Quality of Life in Patients with Breast Cancer Receiving Endocrine Therapy?[88]

Women's vasomotor symptoms were reduced with the investigational drug, elinzanetant.

Women receiving endocrine therapy for the treatment or prevention of breast cancer commonly report vasomotor symptoms. Current treatments (gabapentin, low-dose antidepressants, acupuncture, lifestyle interventions, and complementary products like black cohosh) have not been very effective. In an industry-supported, phase 3 study, Cardoso et al. examined the effectiveness of the investigational drug elinzanetant in 474 women with moderate-to-severe vasomotor symptoms who were receiving endocrine therapy to treat or prevent breast cancer. Elinzanetant is a neurokinin (NK)-targeted therapy that specifically antagonizes NK-1 and NK-3 receptors, which are implicated in declining estrogenic activity that occurs with natural menopause or antiestrogen medications.

Participants were randomly assigned to once daily elinzanetant for 52 weeks or placebo for 12 weeks, followed by elinzanetant for 40 weeks. At baseline, they experienced a mean of about 11.5 daily moderate-to-severe vasomotor symptoms. At week 4, women taking elinzanetant experienced a significantly greater drop in symptoms than women on placebo (mean change, −6.5 vs. −3.0 episodes). The results remained significant at week 12 (−7.8 vs. −4.2 episodes). Elinzanetant was associated with improved sleep and quality of life. Most adverse events were mild or moderate. Somnolence, fatigue, and diarrhea were more frequent with elinzanetant than placebo through week 12. More than 90% of participants chose to continue elinzanetant through the 2-year extension.

Switch to a SERD Before Clinical Progression in *ESR1*-Mutated Advanced Breast Cancer?[91]

For patients with advanced breast cancer who acquire ESR1 mutations during first-line aromatase inhibitor (AI) and CDK4/6 inhibitor therapy, switching to camizestrant — before disease progression — improves PFS.

In early trials, camizestrant, a next-generation selective estrogen receptor degrader (SERD) and complete ER antagonist, demonstrated activity in patients with ESR1-mutated breast cancer. A strategy to change systemic therapy based on molecular evolution of the cancer before clinical evidence of progression has been considered a means to improve survival, but has not yet been convincingly proven.

In the industry-funded, phase 3 SERENA-6 trial, nearly 3,300 patients with ER+/HER2− advanced breast cancer who had received at least 6 months of first-line treatment with an aromatase inhibitor plus a CDK4/6 inhibitor, and did not have evidence of disease progression, underwent testing for ESR1 mutations in circulating tumor DNA every 2 to 3 months. Ultimately, 315 patients who tested positive for ESR1 mutations were randomized either to switch to camizestrant plus a CDK4/6 inhibitor (plus a placebo AI) or to continue an AI plus a CDK4/6 inhibitor (plus placebo in place of camizestrant).

During a median follow-up of roughly 13 months, progression-free survival (PFS) — the primary end point — favored the camizestrant group (median, 16.0 months, vs. 9.2 months in the AI group). The estimated percentage of patients who were alive without progression at 24 months was 30% versus 5%, respectively.

Grade 3 or higher adverse events occurred in 60% of the camizestrant group and 46% of the AI group. Hematologic events accounted for most of this difference.

The SERENA-6 study may represent a paradigm shift in how oncologists manage patients with ER+/HER2− metastatic breast cancer without clinical or radiologic evidence of disease progression while receiving an AI and CDK4/6 inhibitor. If an ESR1 mutation emerges before clinical evidence of recurrence, switching the AI to the SERD camizestrant significantly extends PFS.

Respiratory Infections Can Awaken Breast Cancer Metastases[67]

COVID-19 or influenza infections were associated with higher risk for lung metastases in cancer survivors.

An international team reported that, in mice, infection with either influenza virus or SARS-CoV-2 causes a >100-fold expansion of lung metastases within 2 weeks. The transition is dependent on the proinflammatory cytokine, interleukin-6 (IL-6), which activates the JAK-STAT signalling pathway. The disseminated cancer cells then "teach" CD4+ T cells to inhibit the CD8+ T cell response mounted against cancer cell proliferation.

When these researchers retrospectively studied nearly 37,000 women with known breast cancer, the chance of newly observed pulmonary metastases was 1.4 times higher in those who received COVID-19 diagnoses than in those who did not. Among nearly 5,000 people with cancer of any type in remission, those who were infected by SARS-CoV-2 were 2.6 times more likely to die from cancer subsequently than those who were not infected, after multivariate adjustment. Risk was greatest shortly after infections and decreased over time.

Does Risk-Reducing Surgery Benefit Young Breast Cancer Survivors with *BRCA* Mutations?[96]

Patients 40 and younger who underwent bilateral salpingo-oophorectomy and bilateral mastectomy had significantly longer overall survival.

For carriers of BRCA1 or BRCA2 mutations, it has long been known that bilateral salpingo-oophorectomy (BSO) and bilateral mastectomy reduce cancer risk in those organs. Similarly, for patients with BRCA mutations who develop breast cancer and undergo risk-reducing BSO (RRBSO), breast cancer–related survival is improved. In this study researchers retrospectively studied an international cohort of >5,000 young patients (≤40 years) who received a diagnosis of stage I–III breast cancer from 2000 to 2020 to determine the effect of such surgery on overall survival.

Patients could have undergone breast-conserving surgery or mastectomy as primary surgical therapy for the initial breast cancer. Overall, 64% of patients were BRCA1 pathogenic variant carriers, 51% had node-negative disease, and 46% had hormone-receptor–positive disease; 55% underwent risk-reducing mastectomy (RRM), 53% underwent RRBSO, and 34% underwent both.

Median follow-up was 8 years. Patients who underwent RRM had significantly longer estimated overall survival at 20 years after breast cancer diagnosis than those who did not undergo RRM (average,17.9 vs. 16.7 years). RRBSO was also associated with a significant overall survival benefit compared with no RRBSO (average, 17.7 vs. 16.7 years).

During the 20-year study period, changes in the indications for germline genetic testing and the introduction of new treatments — such as PARP inhibitors and CDK4/6 inhibitors — could have affected outcomes in patients most recently added to the overall cohort. Regardless, risk-reduction surgery clearly confers a survival benefit for young patients with BRCA mutations and a prior diagnosis of breast cancer.

Does Hormonal Contraception Influence Breast Cancer Risk?[101]

When counselling patients about hormonal contraception, it should be stated that a small excess breast cancer risk is associated with most options. It can be helpful to note that combined oral contraceptives have benefits in reducing risk of ovarian, endometrial, and colorectal cancers, and that levonorgestrel intrauterine systems can reduce the risk of endometrial cancer. For those at high risk for breast cancer, it seems sensible to focus on the options with no observed excess risk in this study: the vaginal ring, drospirenone-based combinations, or depot medroxyprogesterone acetate.

Hormonal contraceptive options carry a small excess risk for breast cancer, but it is unclear whether the risk varies by contraceptive type, duration of use, and route of administration. To address this gap, researchers assessed risk for breast cancer associated with hormonal contraceptive use in a cohort of Swedish adolescents and women (ages 13–49) and followed them for up to 13 years (until the end of the study or age 50, whichever came first).

Among 2 million women, there were 16,385 cases of breast cancer.

Use of hormonal contraceptives was linked to a very small excess risk (roughly 13 additional cases per 100,000 users per year). Risk increased with duration of use.

Excess risk was similar across most contraceptive methods. The largest relative increase was observed with desogestrel-containing combined pills (hazard ratio,

1.19), progestin-only desogestrel pills (HR, 1.18), and the etonogestrel implant (HR, 1.22), though the absolute increase in risk remained low. Several methods (drospirenone-containing combined pills, depot medroxyprogesterone acetate injection, and the etonogestrel vaginal ring) showed no measurable excess risk.

Statin Use Might Affect Breast Cancer Survival[149]

Statin drugs inhibit the mevalonate pathway, which is essential not only for cholesterol production but also for cancer cell proliferation, survival, and metastases. In a Danish registry study of 67,000 women with stage I to III breast cancer (diagnosed with between 2000 and 2021) and without prior statin exposure, researchers evaluated associations between statin initiation after breast cancer diagnosis and mortality. Patients were followed for 10 years or until death.

- Women who initiated statins within 3 years after breast cancer diagnosis had significantly lower 10-year breast cancer–related mortality than did non-initiators (11.8% vs. 13.5%; hazard ratio, 0.9).
- All-cause mortality also was lower with statin initiation, but this finding did not meet prespecified statistical significance (HR, 0.92; 95% confidence interval, 0.85–1.00).
- Starting statins closer to the time of diagnosis had more favorable effects with significant risk reductions for both breast cancer-related and all-cause mortality.
- Five-year overall survival was significantly better among statin initiators (89.8% vs 87.8%).

This study's design emulated the Mammary Cancer Statin ER Positive (MASTER) study, an ongoing randomized, placebo-controlled, phase 3 trial in which researchers are examining the benefits of adding atorvastatin to standard adjuvant therapy in women with early breast cancer. Despite this observational study's careful design, residual confounding is possible, and causality cannot be determined. If the results from MASTER are favorable, adjuvant statin treatment could be valuable in this population.

Is Postmastectomy Radiation Necessary for Intermediate-Risk Breast Cancer?[109]

No survival benefit was seen in the latest international trial.

Postmastectomy radiation therapy reduces local recurrence risk and prolongs survival in patients at high risk for breast cancer recurrence, including those with a high nodal burden, but the situation is less clear for those at intermediate risk for recurrence.To address this, investigators conducted an international, phase 3, randomized trial (SUPREMO) comparing chest-wall radiation with no radiation therapy in 1600 women who had undergone mastectomy for intermediate-risk breast cancer.

Approximately 30% of the women had stage T1N1 disease; 25% had T2N0 disease with grade 3 histology, lymphovascular invasion, or both; and 45% had T2N1 disease. Roughly 85% received chemotherapy (which consisted of anthracycline-based regimens, with or without a taxane), 80% received endocrine therapy, and 20% received trastuzumab. The median follow-up was 9.6 years.

- Both treatment groups had a 10-year survival rate of 81%. Disease-free survival (76%) and distant metastasis–free survival (78%) were also similar between the groups.
- Intermediate-risk patients derived no benefit from postmastectomy radiation therapy in this trial — perhaps because systemic therapy has become so effective as to render radiation unnecessary among patients with intermediate-risk breast cancer.

The authors acknowledged that advances in systemic therapy may explain why the mortality rate was lower than expected in this trial, as was the number of chest-wall recurrences. Taken together, these findings suggest that with today's systemic therapies, radiation therapy can be de-escalated in patients with intermediate-risk breast cancer, sparing them unnecessary toxicity without compromising survival outcomes

Vepdegestrant, a PROTAC Estrogen Receptor Degrader, in Advanced Breast Cancer[150]

Among patients with ER-positive, HER2-negative advanced breast cancer, vepdegestrant was associated with significantly longer progression-free survival than fulvestrant in the subgroup with ESR1 mutations but not in the full patient population.

Vepdegestrant is an oral proteolysis-targeting chimera (PROTAC) estrogen receptor (ER) degrader that directly harnesses the ubiquitin–proteasome system.

In this phase 3, open-label, randomized trial, the investigators enrolled patients with ER-positive, human epidermal growth factor receptor 2 (HER2)–negative advanced breast cancer who had received one previous line of cyclin-dependent kinase 4 and 6 inhibitor therapy plus one line of endocrine therapy (and up to one additional line of endocrine therapy). Patients were randomly assigned in a 1:1 ratio to receive vepdegestrant at a dose of 200 mg orally once every day of each 28-day cycle or fulvestrant at a dose of 500 mg, administered intramuscularly, on day 1 and day 15 of cycle 1 and on day 1 of subsequent cycles, with randomization stratified according to ESR1-mutation status and presence or absence of visceral disease. [Fulvestrant is a selective estrogen receptor degrader (SERD) and was first-in-class to be approved. It works by binding to the estrogen receptor and destabilizing it, causing the cell's normal protein degradation processes to destroy it]. The primary end point was progression-free survival as assessed by blinded independent central review among the patients with ESR1 mutations and among all the patients who underwent randomization. Progression-free survival was estimated with Kaplan–Meier methods and hazard ratios with a stratified Cox proportional-hazards model.

A total of 624 patients underwent randomization; 313 were assigned to receive vepdegestrant, and 311 to receive fulvestrant. Among the 270 patients with ESR1 mutations, the median progression-free survival was 5.0 months (95% confidence interval [CI], 3.7 to 7.4) with vepdegestrant and 2.1 months (95% CI, 1.9 to 3.5) with fulvestrant (hazard ratio, 0.58 [95% CI, 0.43 to 0.78]; $P<0.001$). Among all the patients, the median progression-free survival was 3.8 months (95% CI, 3.7 to 5.3) with vepdegestrant and 3.6 months (95% CI, 2.6 to 4.0) with fulvestrant (hazard ratio, 0.83 [95% CI, 0.69 to 1.01]; $P=0.07$). Adverse events of grade 3 or higher occurred in 23.4% of the patients in the vepdegestrant group and in 17.6% of the patients in the fulvestrant group. Adverse events led to treatment discontinuation in 2.9% and 0.7% of the patients, respectively.

Sacituzumab Govitecan in Untreated, Advanced Triple-Negative Breast Cancer[113]

Patients with previously untreated, locally advanced, unresectable or metastatic triple-negative breast cancer who are not candidates for inhibitors of programmed cell death protein 1 (PD-1) or programmed death ligand 1 (PD-L1) have limited treatment options.

In this international, phase 3, open-label, randomized trial, the investigators enrolled patients with previously untreated, advanced triple-negative breast cancer who were not candidates for PD-1 or PD-L1 inhibitors owing to previous use or coexisting conditions. Patients had either PD-L1–negative tumors with a combined positive score (CPS; the number of PD-L1–staining tumor cells, lymphocytes, and macrophages divided by the total number of viable tumor cells, multiplied by 100) of less than 10 or PD-L1–positive tumors with a CPS of 10 or higher and were assigned in a 1:1 ratio to receive sacituzumab govitecan or chemotherapy (paclitaxel, nanoparticle albumin-bound paclitaxel, or gemcitabine plus carboplatin). The primary end point was progression-free survival, assessed by blinded independent central review. Secondary end points included overall survival, objective response, the duration of response, and safety.

Among 558 patients, median progression-free survival was 9.7 months (95% confidence interval [CI], 8.1 to 11.1) with sacituzumab govitecan and 6.9 months (95% CI, 5.6 to 8.2) with chemotherapy (stratified hazard ratio for disease progression or death, 0.62; 95% CI, 0.50 to 0.77; $P<0.001$). An objective response was confirmed in 48% of patients (95% CI, 42 to 54) who received sacituzumab govitecan and 46% (95% CI, 40 to 52) who received chemotherapy. The median response duration was 12.2 months (95% CI, 9.7 to 13.8) and 7.2 months (95% CI, 5.7 to 8.4), respectively. Adverse events of grade 3 or higher occurred in 66% of patients who received sacituzumab govitecan (most frequently neutropenia [in 43%], diarrhea [in 9%], and leukopenia [in 7%]) and in 62% of patients who received chemotherapy (most frequently neutropenia [in 41%], anemia [in 16%], and leukopenia [in 13%]). The incidence of adverse events that led to discontinuation of sacituzumab govitecan or at least one chemotherapy drug was 4% and 12%, respectively.

Sacituzumab govitecan led to significantly longer progression-free survival than chemotherapy among patients with advanced triple-negative breast cancer who were not candidates for treatment with PD-1 or PD-L1 inhibitors. The incidence of adverse events of grade 3 or higher with sacituzumab govitecan was similar to that with chemotherapy, but adverse events were common.

Ten-Year Survival after Postmastectomy Chest-Wall Irradiation in Breast Cancer[114]

In this trial, chest-wall irradiation did not result in higher overall survival than no chest-wall irradiation among patients with intermediate-risk, early breast cancer treated with mastectomy and contemporary adjuvant systemic therapy.

The role of postmastectomy chest-wall irradiation in patients with breast cancer classified as pN1 (with involvement of one to three axillary nodes) or pN0 (pathologically node negative) with additional risk factors is uncertain.

In this international, phase 3, randomized trial, the investigators evaluated the omission of chest-wall irradiation in women with “intermediate-risk” breast cancer - defined as cancer that was stage pT1N1, pT2N1, or pT3N0 or stage pT2N0 with a histologic grade of 3, lymphovascular invasion, or both (tumor size: T1, ≤2 cm; T2, >2 cm to 5 cm; or T3, >5 cm) - that was treated with mastectomy, an axillary procedure, and systemic therapy. Patients were assigned to undergo chest-wall irradiation (40 to 50 Gy; the irradiation group) or not to undergo chest-wall irradiation (the no-irradiation group). The primary end point was overall survival, with 10 years of follow-up. Chest-wall recurrence, regional recurrence, disease-free survival, distant metastasis–free survival, causes of death, and radiation-related adverse events were also assessed.

The intention-to-treat population included 808 patients in the irradiation group and 799 in the no-irradiation group. The median follow up was 9.6 years. Overall survival was 81.4% with chest-wall irradiation and 81.9% with no chest-wall irradiation according to 10-year Kaplan–Meier estimates (hazard ratio for death, 1.04; 95% confidence interval [CI], 0.82 to 1.30; P=0.80). A total of 29 patients had a chest-wall recurrence - 9 (1.1%) in the irradiation group and 20 (2.5%) in the no-irradiation group (between-group difference, <2 percentage points; hazard ratio, 0.45; 95% CI, 0.20 to 0.99). Disease-free survival was 76.2% in the irradiation group and 75.5% in the no-irradiation group (hazard ratio for recurrence or death, 0.97; 95% CI, 0.79 to 1.18), and distant metastasis–free survival was 78.2% and 79.2%, respectively (hazard ratio for distant metastasis or death, 1.06; 95% CI, 0.86 to 1.31).

In this trial, chest-wall irradiation did not result in higher overall survival than no chest-wall irradiation among patients with intermediate-risk, early breast cancer treated with mastectomy and contemporary adjuvant systemic therapy.

Trastuzumab Deruxtecan plus Pertuzumab for HER2-Positive Metastatic Breast Cancer[121]

Trastuzumab deruxtecan has shown efficacy in patients with previously treated human epidermal growth factor receptor 2 (HER2)–positive advanced or metastatic breast cancer. Trastuzumab deruxtecan plus pertuzumab led to a significantly lower risk of progression or death than taxane, trastuzumab, and pertuzumab (*THP) when used as first-line treatment for HER2-positive advanced or metastatic breast cancer, with no new safety signals.*

The investigators conducted a phase 3 trial involving patients with HER2-positive advanced or metastatic breast cancer and no previous chemotherapy or HER2-directed therapy for metastatic disease. Patients were randomly assigned in a 1:1:1 ratio to receive trastuzumab deruxtecan plus pertuzumab; trastuzumab deruxtecan plus placebo; or a taxane, trastuzumab, and pertuzumab (THP). The primary end point was progression-free survival as assessed by blinded independent central review. Secondary end points included objective response, duration of response, and safety.

For this prespecified interim analysis, data for trastuzumab deruxtecan plus pertuzumab and for THP were reported; data for trastuzumab deruxtecan plus placebo remain blinded until the final analysis of progression-free survival. At the data-cutoff date (February 26, 2025), the median progression-free survival was 40.7 months with trastuzumab deruxtecan plus pertuzumab (383 patients) and 26.9 months with THP (387 patients) (hazard ratio for progression or death, 0.56; 95% confidence interval [CI], 0.44 to 0.71; P<0.00001 [P-value boundary for superiority, 0.00043]). The incidence of a confirmed response was 85.1% with trastuzumab deruxtecan plus pertuzumab and 78.6% with THP (complete responses in 15.1% and 8.5%, respectively), with a median duration of response of 39.2 months and 26.4

months. Safety was consistent with the known profiles of the individual treatments. The incidence of grade 3 or higher adverse events was 63.5% with trastuzumab deruxtecan plus pertuzumab and 62.3% with THP; the most common were neutropenia, hypokalemia, and anemia with trastuzumab deruxtecan plus pertuzumab and neutropenia, leukopenia, and diarrhea with THP. Adjudicated drug-related interstitial lung disease or pneumonitis occurred in 12.1% of patients receiving trastuzumab deruxtecan plus pertuzumab (grade 1 or 2 in 44 patients and grade 5 [death] in 2 patients) and in 1.0% of those receiving THP (all grade 1 or

Trastuzumab deruxtecan plus pertuzumab led to a significantly lower risk of progression or death than THP when used as first-line treatment for HER2-positive advanced or metastatic breast cancer, with no new safety signals.

Omitting Regional Nodal Irradiation after Response to Neoadjuvant Chemotherapy[132]

The addition of adjuvant regional nodal irradiation did not decrease the risk of invasive breast cancer recurrence or death from breast cancer in patients who had negative axillary nodes after neoadjuvant chemotherapy.

The benefit of regional nodal irradiation in the treatment of breast cancer is well established for patients with pathologically positive axillary nodes, but whether it is also beneficial for patients whose nodes become pathologically tumor free (ypN0) after neoadjuvant chemotherapy remains unclear.

The investigators evaluated whether regional nodal irradiation improves outcomes in patients with biopsy-proven, node-positive breast cancer who reach ypN0 status after neoadjuvant chemotherapy. Patients with breast cancer with a clinical stage of T1 to T3 (tumor size, ≤2 cm to >5 cm), N1, and M0 (indicating spread to movable, ipsilateral level I and II axillary lymph nodes but no distant metastasis) who had ypN0 status after neoadjuvant chemotherapy were randomly assigned to receive regional nodal irradiation or no regional nodal irradiation. The primary end point was the interval of freedom from invasive breast cancer recurrence or death from breast cancer (invasive breast cancer recurrence–free interval). Secondary end points included the locoregional recurrence–free interval, the distant recurrence–free interval, disease-free survival, and overall survival. Safety was also assessed.

A total of 1641 patients were enrolled in the trial; 1556 were included in the primary-event analysis: 772 in the irradiation group and 784 in the no-irradiation group. After a median follow-up of 59.5 months, 109 primary end-point events (50 in the irradiation group and 59 in the no-irradiation group) had occurred. Regional nodal irradiation did not significantly increase the invasive breast cancer recurrence–free interval (hazard ratio, 0.88; 95% confidence interval, 0.60 to 1.28; P=0.51). Point estimates of survival free from the primary end-point events were 92.7% in the irradiation group and 91.8% in the no-irradiation group. Regional nodal irradiation did not increase the locoregional recurrence–free interval, the distant recurrence–free interval, disease-free survival, or overall survival. No deaths related to the protocol-specified therapy were reported, and no unexpected adverse events were observed. Grade 4 adverse events occurred in 0.5% of patients in the irradiation group and 0.1% of those in the no-irradiation group.

The addition of adjuvant regional nodal irradiation did not decrease the risk of invasive breast cancer recurrence or death from breast cancer in patients who had negative axillary nodes after neoadjuvant chemotherapy.

Comparing Supplemental Imaging Modalities in Women with Dense Breasts[137]

In a randomized trial, MRI and contrast-enhanced mammography detected more cancers than did ultrasound.

Screening mammography has lower sensitivity among women with dense breasts, but data on supplemental imaging techniques are limited. In this U.K.-based trial, researchers evaluated cancer detection in 6300 middle-aged women (age range, 50–70), who had heterogeneously or extremely dense breasts and negative baseline mammography findings. Participants were randomized to receive one of the following: Abbreviated contrast-enhanced magnetic resonance imaging (MRI); automated whole-breast ultrasound (ABUS), which uses an automated, rather than hand-held, transducer; or iodinated contrast-enhanced mammography.

Cancer-detection rates were 17, 4, and 19 per 1000 women who received MRI, ABUS, and contrast-enhanced mammography, respectively. In contrast, the rate among an observational cohort of women with dense breasts who received mammography alone was 8 per 1000. The average size of detected invasive cancers was smaller for MRI and contrast-enhanced mammography than for ABUS

(≈10 mm vs. 22 mm). MRI and contrast-enhanced mammography had higher recall rates (9.7 per 1000 women), versus 4.0 per 1000 for ABUS. Twenty-eight adverse events (extravasations and contrast reactions) occurred in the MRI and contrast-enhanced mammography groups.

Abbreviated MRI and contrast-enhanced mammography seemingly can detect cancers, including small and early-stage cancers, that would be missed by mammography alone or mammography plus ABUS. However, they also led to more false-positive results and adverse events. Although these findings are intriguing, the survival benefit for cancer detected in this way has not been established; moreover, these modalities are not available widely and generally are not covered by insurance for screening.

De-Escalation of Breast Surgery: Less Is More[3]

Patients with early-stage breast cancer who have ER-positive tumors and clinically node-negative axilla can forego sentinel lymph node biopsy without negative consequence.

Surgical management of early-stage breast cancer has evolved over the last two decades towards de-escalation. Surgeries have become less extensive and the question of whether any surgical intervention is needed for the axilla remains an open question.

In a prospective, noninferiority INSEMA trial, women with clinical stage T1 or T2 tumors, clinical axillary node–negative disease (both by exam and imaging with ultrasound), and a plan for breast-conserving surgery were randomized (1:4) to treatment without axillary surgery or to sentinel lymph node biopsy (SLNB). Patients undergoing SLNB found to have 1 to 3 macrometastases were further randomized to completion axillary dissection or no further axillary surgery (data not mature).

Among the per-protocol population of 4,858 patients, 90% had clinical stage T1 tumors and 79% had surgically confirmed pathological T1 tumors. Approximately 98% of tumors were ER-positive and only 3.6% were HER2-positive. Postoperative adjuvant therapy was similar between groups, except slightly more patients in the surgery group received chemotherapy.

With a median follow-up of 73.6 months, the omission of SLNB was noninferior to surgery for the primary endpoint of 5-year invasive disease-free survival (91.9% and 91.7%). Incidence of axillary recurrence was 1.0% versus 0.3%, respectively, and incidence of death from any cause was1.4% versus 2.4%. Patients not undergoing SLNB had less arm edema/pain and greater arm/shoulder mobility.

The INSEMA study, along with findings from other trials, confirmed that SLNB can be avoided without compromise in local recurrence or survival in patients with clinical T1/T2, ER-positive tumors and clinically node-negative axilla. Since this profile fits an enormous subset of patients with early-stage breast cancer, applying these findings will result in de-escalation of treatment, decreases in therapy-related morbidity, and no compromise in outcome.

Expanding Oral Therapy Options for ER+ Advanced Breast Cancer[11]

The selective estrogen-receptor degrader imlunestrant improved progression-free survival compared with endocrine therapy.

The development of new oral selective estrogen-receptor degraders (SERDs) has increased the treatment options for metastatic ER+/HER2− breast cancer. Imlunestrant is a brain-penetrant SERD shown to have clinical activity in endocrine-refractory tumors, including those that develop ESR1 mutations. It is not yet FDA approved.

In an open-label, phase 3 EMBER-3 trial, 874 patients with ER+/HER2− metastatic breast cancer were randomized to standard of care endocrine therapy (SOC; fulvestrant or exemestane), imlunestrant monotherapy, or imlunestrant plus abemaciclib. Eligible patients had disease progression during or within 12 months after neoadjuvant or adjuvant treatment with an aromatase inhibitor (with or without a CDK4/6 inhibitor), or while receiving first-line treatment.

The median progression-free survival (PFS) was longer with imlunestrant monotherapy than with SOC among patients with ESR1 mutations (5.5 vs. 3.8 months; $P<0.001$) but not among the overall population (5.6 and 5.5 months, respectively; NS). The median PFS with imlunestrant–abemaciclib was longer than with imlunestrant monotherapy (9.4 vs. 5.5 months; $P<0.001$); the improvement with combination therapy was observed whether or not ESR1 mutation was present.

Overall survival was too immature to comment on. (Abemaciclib is a cyclin-dependent kinase inhibitor).

Grade 3 or higher toxicities occurred in roughly 20% of patients in the imlunestrant monotherapy and SOC groups, compared with almost 50% of those receiving combination therapy.

Imlunestrant is active as monotherapy in patients with ESR1 mutations, whereas the combination of imlunestrant and abemaciclib has significant activity in a broader population, including those without ESR1 mutations, but is associated with greater toxicity. The oral SERD elacestrant was recently FDA-approved for patients with ESR1 mutations and is being evaluated in combination with targeted therapies, as are other oral SERDs. If FDA-approved, imlunestrant will be another oral option for patients with ER-positive, metastatic breast cancer.

Triplet Therapy for Bad-Acting ER+ Breast Cancer[17]

Combining endocrine therapy with a CDK4/6 inhibitor and a PIK3CA inhibitor improves outcomes in patients with ER+/HER2− metastatic breast cancer and PIK3CA mutations.

The typical first-line treatment for ER+/HER2− metastatic breast cancer — an endocrine agent combined with a CDK4/6 inhibitor — affords a progression-free survival (PFS) benefit over endocrine therapy alone, but the magnitude of benefit appears to be smaller in the roughly 40% of patients whose tumors harbor PIK3CA mutations. For patients with PIK3CA mutations and disease progression in the first-line setting, combining fulvestrant with either a PI3K inhibitor or an AKT pathway inhibitor for the next treatment provides longer PFS than endocrine therapy alone. Based on these findings, investigators in this study examined whether combining endocrine therapy with a CDK4/6 inhibitor and a PI3K inhibitor could improve outcomes in patients with these more aggressive tumors.

In a phase 3 trial, 325 patients with PIK3CA-mutated, ER+/HER2− metastatic breast cancer were randomly assigned to receive first-line treatment with either inavolisib (an oral selective PI3Kα inhibitor) or placebo, plus fulvestrant and palbociclib. Patients had poor prognostic features, including disease recurrence or progression during or within 12 months after adjuvant endocrine therapy (100%), metastases in at least three organs (≈50%), and liver metastases (≈50%). The median PFS was approximately twice as long in the inavolisib group as in the placebo group (15.0 vs. 7.3 months). Objective response was more frequent with inavolisib than placebo (58.4% vs. 25.0%). Hyperglycemia, a class effect of PI3K inhibitors, occurred in approximately 60% of patients, but grade 3 or 4 hyperglycemia, stomatitis, and diarrhea each occurred in ≤6%.

The triplet combination of an endocrine agent with a CDK4/6 inhibitor and the PI3Kα inhibitor inavolisib improved PFS in a group of patients who tend not to gain as much benefit from the doublet combination of endocrine therapy and a CDK4/6 inhibitor. The behavior of tumors treated with the triplet therapy will need to be assessed post-progression, and determining if an overall survival benefit is derived will be important.

Survival with Trastuzumab Emtansine in Residual HER2-Positive Breast Cancer[22]

The risk of invasive breast cancer or death was 50% lower with adjuvant trastuzumab emtansine (T-DM1) than with trastuzumab alone in patients with HER2–positive early breast cancer who had residual invasive disease after neoadjuvant systemic therapy.

Patients with human epidermal growth factor receptor 2 (HER2)–positive early breast cancer with residual invasive disease after neoadjuvant systemic therapy have a high risk of recurrence and death.

In this study, investigators randomly assigned patients with HER2-positive early breast cancer with residual invasive disease in the breast or axilla after neoadjuvant systemic treatment with taxane-based chemotherapy and trastuzumab to receive T-DM1 or trastuzumab for 14 cycles. They reported the prespecified final analysis of invasive disease–free survival and the second interim analysis of overall survival.

With a median follow-up of 8.4 years, T-DM1 sustained the improvement in invasive disease–free survival over trastuzumab (unstratified hazard ratio for invasive disease or death, 0.54; 95% confidence interval [CI], 0.44 to 0.66). Seven-year invasive disease–free survival was 80.8% with T-DM1 and 67.1% with trastuzumab (difference, 13.7 percentage points). T-DM1 also led to a significantly lower risk of death than trastuzumab (unstratified hazard ratio, 0.66; 95% CI, 0.51 to 0.87; P=0.003). Seven-year overall survival was 89.1% with T-DM1 and 84.4% with trastuzumab (difference, 4.7 percentage points). Adverse events of grade 3 or higher were noted in 26.1% of the patients in the T-DM1 group and 15.7% of those in the trastuzumab group.

As compared with trastuzumab, T-DM1 improved overall survival with sustained improvement in invasive disease–free survival among patients with HER2-positive early breast cancer with residual invasive disease after neoadjuvant therapy.

De-Escalation of Surgery in Ductal Carcinoma In Situ (DCIS)[53]

In women with low-risk DCIS, incidence of ipsilateral invasive cancer was not higher with active monitoring compared with guideline-concordant care.

The noninferiority COMET trial compared outcomes between patients randomized to current guideline-concordant care (surgery with or without radiation therapy) or active monitoring without surgical intervention (breast imaging and physical exam every 6 months). Eligible participants were women aged 40 years and older with newly diagnosed, screen-detected, nuclear grade 1 or 2 ER/PR-positive, HER2-negative DCIS.

Of 997 women enrolled, 75% were white and 16% Black. At diagnosis, 75% had grade II DCIS and 25% grade 1. With a median follow-up of 37 months, 264 women in the guideline-concordant group and 82 in the active monitoring group underwent surgery. Ipsilateral invasive cancer was diagnosed in 27 women in the guideline-concordant group and 19 in the active-monitoring group. The 2-year cumulative rate of ipsilateral invasive cancer – the primary outcome — was 5.9% versus 4.2%, respectively; this result met the noninferiority threshold, thereby demonstrating short-term safety of active monitoring.

The COMET study is important but needs to be validated by other ongoing studies.

Postoperative Checkpoint Inhibitors for Early-Stage Triple-Negative Breast Cancer?[33]

The addition of atezolizumab to adjuvant chemotherapy did not improve outcomes compared with chemotherapy alone.

Immunotherapy improves outcomes for patients with early-stage triple-negative breast cancer (TNBC), but how to optimally use it and in which patients remain open questions. The KEYNOTE-522 trial showed that the addition of pembrolizumab to preoperative chemotherapy increased pathological complete response rate and improved event-free and overall survival (NEJM JW Oncol Hematol Feb 11 2022 and N Engl J Med 2022; 386:556). Trial participants continued pembrolizumab postoperatively, although the contribution of the postoperative component to overall outcome is still debated.

There are patients who undergo surgery as a first step, either by design or because they do not meet the eligibility criteria for the KEYNOTE-522 regimen, but their pathology results suggest they may have been appropriate candidates for the regimen. Would postoperative immunotherapy confer benefit in this situation?

These investigators reported results from the phase 3 ALEXANDRA/IMpassion030 study in which 2,199 patients with stage II or III TNBC who underwent surgery as the initial treatment were randomized postoperatively to standard adjuvant chemotherapy or chemotherapy plus the checkpoint inhibitor atezolizumab for up to 1 year. The primary endpoint was invasive disease-free survival.

Patients' median age was 53 years, 52% were node negative, and 35% had 1 to 3 involved nodes. At surgery, 85% had stage II disease, 15% stage III. With a median follow-up of 32 months, the trial was stopped early after an interim analysis indicated futility. The addition of atezolizumab did not decrease recurrence rates or deaths compared with adjuvant chemotherapy alone. Furthermore, grade 3/4 toxicities were greater with the addition of immunotherapy (54% vs. 44%).

This trial demonstrated no benefit for postoperative immunotherapy in patients with early-stage TNBC who did not receive chemoimmunotherapy in the neoadjuvant setting. Some ongoing clinical trials are exploring postoperative immunotherapy, but at present, immunotherapy should be used as a component of neoadjuvant treatment and continued postoperatively.

Long-Term Cardiac Tolerability of Trastuzumab[151]

Decisions to continue or resume therapy after adverse cardiac events must include evaluation of risks and benefits. This study included patients who had received trastuzumab for at least 1 year. Most patients with trastuzumab-associated cardiac toxicity recovered completely, and many were re-treated with trastuzumab, without additional cardiac toxicity. A substantial number of patients did not discontinue trastuzumab, despite cardiac dysfunction.

Patients who experience trastuzumab-induced cardiac toxicity should be managed in concert with cardiologists, and decisions to continue or resume trastuzumab must be made only after careful discussion of the potential benefits and risks associated with further therapy.

Trastuzumab (Herceptin), a humanized anti-HER2 monoclonal antibody, is highly effective for treating HER2-overexpressing invasive breast cancer. In patients with HER2-positive metastatic breast cancer, trastuzumab plus chemotherapy improved objective response rate, time-to-disease progression, and overall survival, compared with chemotherapy alone. In the pivotal randomized trial, 28% of patients who received trastuzumab plus chemotherapy (predominantly those who received concurrent trastuzumab and anthracycline-based chemotherapy) experienced adverse cardiac events. More recently, in several large randomized clinical trials, trastuzumab in combination with adjuvant chemotherapy has significantly lowered risk for recurrence in patients with early-stage breast cancer. However, the collective experience from adjuvant therapy trials suggests that ~5% of patients who receive trastuzumab will show some evidence of systolic cardiac dysfunction. Follow-up reports suggest that most patients who develop trastuzumab-induced cardiac dysfunction will recover normal cardiac function when trastuzumab is discontinued, with or without subsequent medical management.

Researchers now report on the long-term cardiac status of 173 patients with HER2-positive metastatic breast cancer who were treated with trastuzumab for at least 1 year (median cumulative time of trastuzumab administration, 21.3 months; median follow-up, 33.6 months). Standard clinical practice included cardiac evaluation in which left ventricular ejection fraction (LVEF) and cardiac toxicity were assessed. A total of 49 patients (28%) experienced adverse cardiac events: 3 patients showed asymptomatic decreases (>50%) in LVEF, 27 patients experienced grade 2 cardiac toxicity (LVEF range, 40%–50%), and 19 patients experienced grade 3 cardiac toxicity (symptoms of congestive heart failure (CHF) or LVEF range, 20%–40%). Only 15 patients were symptomatic at diagnosis; one patient with CHF died.

In patients who developed either CHF or large asymptomatic decreases in LVEF, trastuzumab was discontinued. For other patients, decisions to stop or continue therapy were made on a case-by-case basis. Fourteen symptomatic patients discontinued trastuzumab and 11 recovered, with or without cardiac therapy. Among the asymptomatic patients, 17 discontinued trastuzumab, and 15 recovered; 17 continued trastuzumab, and 15 recovered. In 26 patients (symptomatic or asymptomatic) who discontinued therapy, trastuzumab therapy was resumed after complete cardiac recovery: 16 patients experienced no further adverse cardiac events, whereas 10 experienced additional adverse events. Of these 10, 5 recovered completely after trastuzumab was discontinued again, and 5 maintained a slightly lowered LVEF (asymptomatic) while continuing trastuzumab.

Inavolisib in *PIK3CA*-Mutated Advanced Breast Cancer[95]

Adding inavolisib to palbociclib–fulvestrant extended overall survival in certain patients with aggressive disease.

For patients with ER+/HER2− metastatic breast cancer, standard first line therapy is usually an endocrine agent plus an aromatase inhibitor. The subset of patients with tumors harboring a PIK3CA mutation, particularly patients with rapid progression following adjuvant therapy, have a shorter progression-free interval than those with PIK3CA wild-type tumors.

In a phase 3 INAVO120 trial, researchers enrolled 325 adults with locally advanced or metastatic PIK3CA-mutated, hormone receptor–positive, HER2-negative, endocrine-resistant breast cancer who had disease recurrence or progression after completing adjuvant endocrine therapy. Patients were randomized to receive either the selective PI3Kα inhibitor inavolisib (9 mg orally once daily) or placebo; all participants received palbociclib and fulvestrant.

The inavolisib group had a median overall survival of 34 months, compared with 27 months in the placebo group. Progression-free survival (PFS) favored the inavolisib group (median, 17 vs. 7 months for placebo). In addition, the inavolisib group had a significantly greater objective response rate than the placebo group (63% vs. 28%).

Inavolisib recipients had higher incidences of hyperglycemia, stomatitis or mucosal inflammation, diarrhea, and ocular toxicities. They were also more likely to experience serious adverse events (27% vs. 14% of placebo recipients).

The addition of inavolisib to palbociclib–fulvestrant confers not only an improvement in PFS but also, importantly, overall survival for a group of patients who have more aggressive disease (i.e., rapid progression following adjuvant endocrine therapy).

Addressing HER2-Positive Residual Breast Cancer[99]

The survival benefit of adjuvant trastuzumab emtansine over trastuzumab alone was sustained at long-term follow-up in patients with residual disease following neoadjuvant HER2-directed therapy.

It has long been recognized that, among patients with HER2-positive breast cancer receiving neoadjuvant HER2 -directed therapy, those with residual disease at the time of surgery have a worse prognosis than those with a pathologic complete response. Investigators from the open-label, randomized, phase 3 KATHERINE trial previously reported that patients with residual disease after taxane-based HER2-directed neoadjuvant therapy had a 50% reduction in the risk for invasive breast cancer or death at 3 years with adjuvant trastuzumab emtansine (T-DM1) versus adjuvant trastuzumab alone. Now, with a median follow-up of 8.4 years, the investigators reported that the benefit was sustained.

Seven-year invasive disease-free survival was 80.8% with T-DM1 versus 67.1% with trastuzumab, an absolute improvement of 13.7%. Additionally, T-DM1 was associated with a 34% relative reduction in death compared with trastuzumab. 7-year overall survival was 89.1% with T-DM1 versus 84.4% with trastuzumab. No new safety concerns were identified.

COLO-RECTAL CANCER

Adjuvant Therapy for high risk Stage II Colon Cancer[1]

Oxaliplatin adds no overall survival benefit to 6 months of fluorinated pyrimidine chemotherapy for these patients.

Given the relatively low risk of recurrence after resection of stage II colon cancer, treatment guidelines include consideration for observation alone or adjuvant chemotherapy. Patients with stage II disease and features including a T4 primary tumor, presentation with perforation or obstruction, or inadequate lymph sampling at surgery have a higher risk for recurrence and are more strongly considered for adjuvant chemotherapy. The adjuvant treatment of patients with high-risk stage II colon cancer with fluorinated pyrimidine (FP) (such as 5-fluorouracil) alone or with the addition of oxaliplatin remains controversial. The investigators reported an ACCENT database pooled analysis of data from the MOSAIC and C-07 randomized trials comparing 6 months of adjuvant FP-based chemotherapy with oxaliplatin versus without oxaliplatin after resection of stage II and III colon cancer. Of the 1595 patients with stage II disease, 57% had left-sided primaries, 14% had stage T4 cancer, 13% had poorly differentiated tumors, 45% had fewer than 12 lymph nodes sampled at surgery, and 24% presented with perforation or obstruction. Overall survival did not differ between patients treated with FP alone or FP plus oxaliplatin (hazard ratio, 1.03). Overall survival (OS) also did not differ with and without the addition of oxaliplatin in high-risk subgroups including patients with T4 disease (HR, 0.96) and those with fewer than 12 lymph nodes sampled (HR, 0.89). This pooled analysis reinforces the absence of benefit from adding oxaliplatin to 6 months of adjuvant FP chemotherapy in high-risk stage II colon cancer, and one standard of care remains 6 months of FP chemotherapy.

Additionally, a recent pooled analysis of six international, randomized adjuvant therapy trials supported a shorter duration of 3 months of therapy with the combination of capecitabine and oxaliplatin for high-risk stage II disease.

First-Line Immune Checkpoint Inhibitor Therapy for MSI-High Metastatic Colon Cancer[12]

In a randomized trial, 24-month progression-free survival was significantly higher with nivolumab plus ipilimumab than with chemotherapy.

Pembrolizumab achieves superior response, progression-free survival (PFS) and overall survival compared with first-line chemotherapy in patients with microsatellite-instability (MSI)–high metastatic colorectal cancer (CRC). Nonrandomized trials have also indicated a high degree of effectiveness for single-agent nivolumab or the combination of ipilimumab and nivolumab (ipi/nivo).

Investigators reported results of a phase 3 Checkmate 8HW trial comparing treatment with first-line chemotherapy versus ipi/nivo in patients with previously untreated unresectable or metastatic MSI-high CRC. Patients were randomly assigned to treatment with investigators' choice of chemotherapy with or without a targeted agent, or nivolumab (240 mg) and ipilimumab (1 mg/kg) every 3 weeks for 12 weeks, followed by nivolumab maintenance (480 mg) every 4 weeks. Of 303 patients, 68% had right-sided primaries, 39% had liver and 42% had peritoneal metastases, 84% had centrally confirmed MSI-high status, and 13% had known Lynch syndrome.

At a median follow-up of 31.5 months, the primary endpoint of PFS in the patients with centrally confirmed MSI-high status was superior for ipi/nivo compared with chemotherapy ($P<0.001$), both at 12 months (79% vs. 21%) and 24 months (72% vs. 14%). Estimated mean survival time at 24 months was numerically superior for ipi/nivo compared with chemotherapy (19.2 vs. 8.6 months). All subgroups, including patients with RAS and BRAF mutations, achieved superior PFS with ipi/nivo. Treatment-related grade 3/4 serious adverse events were less common with ipi/nivo than chemotherapy (23% vs. 49%). No new safety concerns were observed.

Liver Transplantation plus Chemotherapy vs. Chemotherapy Alone in Metastatic Colorectal Cancer[19]

Selected patients with liver-confined, unresectable disease might benefit from transplantation.

Patients with metastatic colorectal cancer with liver-only metastases benefit from regional therapies, including surgery. The selective application of liver transplantation in these patients is still debated. In this study investigators reported results of the

TransMet trial, which involved patients with unresectable liver-confined, *BRAF* wild-type metastatic colorectal cancer who had achieved stable disease or response to ≥3 months of chemotherapy. Patients were randomized to continue chemotherapy or to undergo liver transplantation followed by additional chemotherapy.

Of the 94 patients enrolled, 15% had right-sided primaries, 32% had *RAS* mutations, nearly 100% presented with synchronous metastases, and 87% achieved either response or stable disease to first-line chemotherapy. The average number of liver metastases was 20, and the average number of treatment cycles at randomization was 21 in the transplant arm and 17 in the chemotherapy arm. Of the 47 transplant-arm patients, 38 (81%) underwent transplantation, and of the 47 chemotherapy-alone patients, 9 (19%) underwent surgical intervention (hepatic resection in 7, and liver transplantations in 2).

The primary endpoint, 5-year overall survival, was superior for transplant versus chemotherapy in the intention-to-treat (56.6% vs. 12.6%) and per-protocol analyses (73.2% vs. 9.3%). Three-year overall survival was 65.5% and 38.9%.

Of the transplant-arm patients who underwent transplantation, 72% experienced metastatic recurrence, largely in the lungs and lymph nodes, and 46% underwent surgery or local ablation, with a secondary progression-free survival rate of 36.1% at 5 years. Transplantation appeared tolerable, with comparable rates of serious adverse events for the transplant and chemotherapy arms (80% and 83%).

Sotorasib plus Panitumumab for Mutated *kras* g12c Metastatic Colon Cancer[22]

This combination resulted in higher PFS and response rates than trifluridine-tipiracil or regorafenib.

Novel inhibitors of mutated *KRAS* G12C, such as sotorasib and adagrasib, have shown efficacy across the spectrum of solid tumors, including non–small-cell lung, colorectal, and pancreatic cancer. Because inhibition of KRAS G12C may be overcome by feedback activation of the EGFR receptor, dual targeting combining an EGFR inhibitor with a KRAS G12C inhibitor has been studied.

In this study investigators reported results of an open-label, phase 3 trial in which patients with mutated *KRAS* G12C metastatic colon cancer were randomized to treatment with oral sotorasib at a dose of 240 mg daily combined with panitumumab

(6 mg/kg IV every two weeks), sotorasib at a dose of 960 mg daily plus panitumumab, or investigators' choice of standard care trifluridine-tipiracil or regorafenib. Of the 160 patients, 66% had colon primaries, 63% had left-sided primaries, and 85% had received two or more prior treatment regimens.

At a median follow-up of 7.8 months, the primary endpoint of progression-free survival (PFS) was superior for sotorasib plus panitumumab at both the 960 mg and 240 mg doses compared to standard care (median, 5.6 and 3.9 vs. 2.2 months; hazard ratios, 0.49 and 0.58, respectively). The response rate was also higher with sotorasib plus panitumumab at 940 mg and 240 mg than with standard care (26.4% and 5.7% vs. 0%). Overall survival data has not matured. Grade 3 or higher treatment-related adverse events included acneiform rash, rash, diarrhea, and hypomagnesemia in the sotorasib arms, and neutropenia, nausea, anemia, and hypertension in the standard care arm.

The combination of sotorasib and panitumumab yielded superior PFS and higher response rates compared to standard care therapy. Results were more favorable with the higher dose of sotorasib, without increased side effects compared with the lower dose. Pending overall survival results, this combination will likely move forward in the treatment of *KRAS* G12C mutant colorectal cancer.

Thermal Ablation or Hepatic Resection for Limited Colorectal Liver Metastases?[34]

Thermal ablation was noninferior to resection for overall survival in this randomized trial.

Hepatic resection of limited liver metastases offers curative potential, but for patients with small volume and limited liver involvement, nonsurgical treatment with thermal ablation can also be considered. An international, open-label, randomized, noninferiority COLLISION trial compared hepatic resection to thermal ablation in patients with colorectal cancer and limited (≤10), small (≤3 cm), potentially resectable hepatic metastases.

Of 296 patients, 25% had right-sided and 75% had left-sided or rectal primaries, 78% received induction chemotherapy, and 67% had unknown or missing *RAS* or *BRAF* mutation status. Limited surgery and limited ablation were permitted in both treatment groups; in the group randomized to surgery, 61% underwent surgery alone and 35% resection plus ablation, and in the group randomized to ablation, 80% underwent ablation alone and 18% ablation plus resection.

The trial was terminated at a median follow up of 28.9 months after a planned interim analysis indicated that the primary endpoint was achieved: the hazard ratio for median OS (1.05) was less than the upper limit of noninferiority (1.3; P=0.81). Overall survival was nearly identical in the thermal ablation and hepatic resection groups at 1 year (93%), 2 years (79%), and 5 years (51% and 55%). Distant progression-free survival was similar in the surgery and thermal ablation groups (median, 8.4 and 9.6 months). Thermal ablation resulted in fewer serious adverse events than resection (7% vs. 20%).

The COLLISION trial provides randomized trial evidence that thermal ablation is noninferior to surgical resection for patients with colorectal cancer with limited hepatic metastases. Thermal ablation can be considered as an alternative first-line option to surgical management in these patients.

Combination or Single-Agent Immune Checkpoint Inhibition in MSI-High/dMMR Metastatic Colorectal Cancer?[36]

Progression-free survival and response rate were superior with the combination of ipilimumab and nivolumab compared with nivolumab alone.

For patients with microsatellite instability (MSI)-high/mismatch repair protein-deficient (dMMR) metastatic colorectal cancer, first-line treatment with the immune checkpoint inhibitors pembrolizumab or nivolumab is superior to chemotherapy (NEJM JW Oncol Hematol Dec 3 2020 and N Engl J Med 2020; 383:2207). The role of dual-targeted versus single-agent immune checkpoint inhibition in these patients, however, remained an unanswered question.

In this study, investigators reported results of the open-label, randomized CheckMate 8HW trial comparing single-agent nivolumab with the combination of ipilimumab and nivolumab. The primary endpoint was progression-free survival (PFS) in patients who had centrally confirmed dMMR/MSI-high metastatic colorectal cancer and were being treated in first or later lines of therapy. Of the 707 patients,

57% had received no prior therapy, 68% had right-sided primary cancers, 14% had confirmed Lynch syndrome, and 82% had central confirmation of MSI-high/dMMR status.

At a median follow-up of 47 months, median PFS was superior with ipilimumab/nivolumab compared with single-agent nivolumab (not reached vs. 39.3 months; hazard ratio, 0.62; P=0.0003). At 36 months, 68% of patients in the combination-therapy arm were free of progression compared with 51% of those in the single-agent nivolumab arm. The response rate was significantly higher with combination therapy than with single-agent nivolumab (71% vs. 58%). No new safety side-effects were observed.

The combination of ipilimumab and nivolumab achieved superior PFS and response compared with single-agent nivolumab and represents a new and arguably preferred standard of care in the first-line treatment of MSH-high/dMMR metastatic colorectal cancer. Overall survival results are pending.

First-Line Encorafenib and Cetuximab in BRAF V600E–Mutant Colon Cancer[44]

Adding encorafenib and cetuximab to first-line chemotherapy significantly improves response rates and duration of response, making it the new standard of care.

In December 2024, the U.S. FDA granted accelerated approval for the combination of encorafenib and cetuximab (EC) with mFOLFOX6 (oxaliplatin, leucovorin, and 5-FU) for first-line treatment of BRAF-mutant colorectal cancer, based on the results of the industry-sponsored, phase 3 BREAKWATER trial. Now, investigators have published results of this trial, which featured dual primary endpoints of objective response rate (ORR) and progression-free survival (PFS).

A total of 479 patients with previously untreated metastatic colorectal cancer with a BRAF V600E mutation were randomized to receive either EC with mFOLFOX6 or standard-of-care chemotherapy. Eighty percent had primary colon cancer, and 61% had right-sided tumors; 52% had prior complete or partial primary tumor resection, and 63% had hepatic metastases. Patients receiving EC and mFOLFOX6 had a significantly greater ORR than those receiving chemotherapy alone (60.9% vs. 40%; odds ratio, 2.4) and a significantly longer median duration of response (13.9 vs. 11.1 months). Data on PFS were not mature at the time of publication, but an interim analysis of overall survival suggested a benefit with EC (hazard ratio, 0.47), although it did not reach statistical significance. Rates of grade 3/4 treatment-related adverse events were higher with EC than with chemotherapy alone (69.7% vs. 53.9%). No new side-effects were observed.

The combination of EC and mFOLFOX6 represents a new first-line standard-of-care therapy in patients with metastatic colorectal cancer with a BRAF V600E mutation.

Aspirin as an Adjuvant Therapy in Colorectal Cancer[59]

Daily aspirin use cuts the risk of colorectal cancer recurrence in half among patients with PIK3CA mutations. These results are practice changing and mandate next-generation sequencing of patients' tumors after curative resection. About 40% of the patients screened for this study harbored somatic PIK3CA mutations, which means that a significant proportion of patients could benefit from taking aspirin after resection.

Aspirin use reduces the risk of colorectal cancer, and retrospective studies have suggested that aspirin use after surgery may reduce recurrence risk, particularly in patients with somatic PIK3CA mutations. Now, investigators report results from a double-blind, randomized, placebo-controlled trial of aspirin use (160 mg daily for 3 years) in 625 patients with resected stage I–III colorectal cancers harboring such mutations. Half had PIK3CA mutations in exon 9 or 20 (group A), and half had other moderate- to high-impact somatic variants in PIK3CA, PIK3R1, or PTEN (group B). About one third had rectal cancer, half had right-sided primary tumors, and a quarter had tumors with high microsatellite instability.

Results were as follows:

- Patients receiving aspirin were half as likely to experience colorectal cancer recurrence by 3 years as those receiving placebo. This was true in group A (14% vs. 8% of patients), group B (17% vs. 8%), and the two combined.
- Subgroup analyses showed significant benefit in patients with rectal cancer and those receiving adjuvant or neoadjuvant therapy. Women appeared to benefit more than men.
- Serious adverse events occurred in 17% of patients receiving aspirin.

Exercise as Medicine for Preventing Colon Cancer Recurrence[73]

Structured exercise significantly reduces recurrence risk and improves survival for stage II and III colon cancer.

While outcomes after surgery and adjuvant chemotherapy for stage II/III colon cancer are generally good, cancer still recurs in about 30% of patients, and quality of life and cardiorespiratory fitness are decreased. Structured exercise improves quality of life and cardiorespiratory outcomes, but conclusive data for cancer outcomes are lacking.

The randomized, phase 3 CHALLENGE trial included nearly 900 patients with high-risk stage II or III colon cancer after completion of adjuvant chemotherapy. Half the patients received a structured, behaviorally supported exercise program over 3 years; the other half received only health-education materials. The primary endpoint was disease-free survival.

Structured exercise notably improved several outcomes compared to education alone:

- 5-year disease-free survival was significantly higher (80.3% vs. 73.9%).
- 8-year overall survival was also significantly higher (90.3% vs. 83.2%).
- Cardiorespiratory fitness showed significantly greater improvement.
- Musculoskeletal adverse events were slightly more common (18.5% vs. 11.5%).

Sustained moderate to vigorous exercise did not just improve quality of life and cardiorespiratory fitness, it yielded a 6–7% absolute improvement in long-term disease-free and overall survival for patients with stage II/III colon cancer — as good or better than adjuvant chemotherapy. The survival improvements were driven by fewer cancer deaths.

Adjuvant Therapy for High-Risk Stage II Colon Cancer[152]

Oxaliplatin added no overall survival benefit to 6 months of fluorinated pyrimidine chemotherapy for these patients.

Given the relatively low risk of recurrence after resection of stage II colon cancer, treatment guidelines include consideration for observation alone or adjuvant chemotherapy. Patients with stage II disease and features including a T4 primary tumor, presentation with perforation or obstruction, or inadequate lymph sampling at surgery have a higher risk for recurrence and are more strongly considered for adjuvant chemotherapy. The adjuvant treatment of patients with high-risk stage II colon cancer with fluorinated pyrimidine (FP) alone or with the addition of oxaliplatin remains controversial.

Investigators reported an ACCENT database pooled analysis of data from the MOSAIC and C-07 randomized trials comparing 6 months of adjuvant FP-based chemotherapy with oxaliplatin versus without oxaliplatin after resection of stage II and III colon cancer. Of the 1595 patients with stage II disease, 57% had left-sided primaries, 14% had stage T4 cancer, 13% had poorly differentiated tumors, 45% had fewer than 12 lymph nodes sampled at surgery, and 24% presented with perforation or obstruction.

Overall survival did not differ between patients treated with FP alone or FP plus oxaliplatin (hazard ratio, 1.03). OS also did not differ with and without the addition of oxaliplatin in high-risk subgroups including patients with T4 disease (HR, 0.96) and those with fewer than 12 lymph nodes sampled (HR, 0.89).

This pooled analysis reinforces the absence of benefit from adding oxaliplatin to 6 months of adjuvant FP chemotherapy in high-risk stage II colon cancer, and one standard of care remains 6 months of FP chemotherapy. The recent pooled IDEA analysis of six international, randomized adjuvant therapy trials supports a shorter duration of 3 months of therapy with the combination of capecitabine and oxaliplatin for high-risk stage II disease (NEJM JW Oncol Hematol Jan 11 2021 and Lancet Oncol 2020; 21:1620).

A Better Treatment for Patients with *BRAF* V600E–Mutant Colon Cancer[94]

Patients had superior overall survival when clinicians added encorafenib and cetuximab to first-line chemotherapy.

In 2024 the FDA granted fast-track approval for the addition of encorafenib and cetuximab to first-line mFOLFOX6 chemotherapy for patients with BRAF V600E–mutant colon cancer based on the combination's superior response rate over chemotherapy alone in the BREAKWATER trial. Investigators now report an update on other endpoints from this open-label, randomized, phase 3 trial.

Patients received one of three treatment combinations:

Encorafenib, cetuximab, and mFOLFOX6 (EC-mFOLFOX6)

Standard-of-care chemotherapy: 5-FU, capecitabine, oxaliplatin, or irinotecan combination therapy with or without bevacizumab (SOC)

Encorafenib and cetuximab without chemotherapy (EC); this arm was closed early.

Of 637 patients, 63% had liver metastases, and 48% had three or more sites of metastases.

Findings for EC-mFOLFOX6 compared with SOC included:

- Median overall survival (OS) was significantly superior (30 months vs. 15 months).
- Median progression-free survival (PFS) showed significant superiority (13 months vs. 7 months).
- Response rate also continued to be superior (66% vs. 37%).

Regarding patients receiving EC, because this arm was discontinued early, statistical analyses were not performed. Nevertheless, the EC patient group had a numerically higher response rate than the SOC group (46%), similar PFS, and a trend toward superior OS (20 months). No new safety signals were observed.

The markedly superior OS for first-line use of EC-mFOLFOX6, along with its superior response and PFS, reinforces this combination as the new standard of care for patients with BRAF V600E–mutant colon cancer.

Combination or Single-Agent Immune Checkpoint Inhibition in MSI-High/dMMR Metastatic Colorectal Cancer?[97]

Progression-free survival and response rate were superior with the combination of ipilimumab and nivolumab compared with nivolumab alone.

For patients with microsatellite instability (MSI)-high/mismatch repair protein-deficient (dMMR) metastatic colorectal cancer, first-line treatment with the immune checkpoint inhibitors pembrolizumab or nivolumab was superior to chemotherapy (NEJM JW Oncol Hematol Dec 3 2020 and N Engl J Med 2020; 383:2207). The role of dual-targeted versus single-agent immune checkpoint inhibition in these patients, however, remained an unanswered question.

Investigators reported results of an open-label, randomized CheckMate 8HW trial comparing single-agent nivolumab with the combination of ipilimumab and nivolumab. The primary endpoint was progression-free survival (PFS) in patients who had centrally confirmed dMMR/MSI-high metastatic colorectal cancer and were being treated in first or later lines of therapy. Of the 707 patients, 57% had received no prior therapy, 68% had right-sided primary cancers, 14% had confirmed Lynch syndrome, and 82% had central confirmation of MSI-high/dMMR status.

At a median follow-up of 47 months, median PFS was superior with ipilimumab/nivolumab compared with single-agent nivolumab (not reached vs. 39.3 months; hazard ratio, 0.62; P=0.0003). At 36 months, 68% of patients in the combination-therapy arm were free of progression compared with 51% of those in the single-agent nivolumab arm. The response rate was significantly higher with combination therapy than with single-agent nivolumab (71% vs. 58%). No new safety signals were observed.

When Does Remission Become a "Cure" in Early-Stage Colon Cancer?[102]

Recurrence rates for stage II and III colon cancer peak 1 year after treatment completion and steadily decline to below 0.5% by 6 years.

Guideline-based surveillance schedules for colon cancer recurrence are derived from large trials and cohort studies but have never been prospectively validated. To determine the point at which remission might be defined as a "cure," researchers examined the timing of recurrence in a pooled analysis of two databases comprising 15 randomized trials; 35,000 patients who had stage II or III cancers (stage III, 83%) and received adjuvant therapy after surgery were included.

- About 27% of patients experienced local or distant recurrences, or both.
- The recurrence rate rose to 6.4% between 6 and 12 months after surgery.

- Recurrence risk then declined continuously, falling below 0.5% by year 6.

This study provided comprehensive data on recurrence risk of stage II and III colorectal cancer. Those who survive to 6 years and are cancer-free are likely cured. Events beyond 6 years are likely second primary tumors or age-related causes of death unrelated to the initial diagnosis. Continuing surveillance with laboratory testing, imaging, or both through 6 years could be beneficial, instead of stopping at 5 years as guidelines currently recommend. Perhaps monitoring circulating tumor DNA could be useful for detecting rare, late recurrences.

Immunotherapy in Late-Line Treatment of Colorectal Cancer[107]

Overall survival was better with zanzalintinib and atezolizumab than with standard-of-care regorafenib.

Multitargeted tyrosine kinase inhibitors (TKIs), including regorafenib, have modest activity in the late-line treatment of metastatic colorectal cancer. Zanzalintinib is an investigational (not FDA-approved) TKI that targets VEGF, TAM kinases (TYRO3, AXL, and MER) and MET. Promising results combining zanzalintinib with the anti–PD-L1 agent atezolizumab prompted the STELLAR-303 trial, an open-label, randomized, phase 3 trial in chemotherapy-refractory colorectal cancer. Patients with microsatellite-stable metastatic colorectal cancer received 100 mg of oral zanzalintinib daily and 1200 mg of atezolizumab intravenously every 3 weeks (ZA) or received standard-of-care treatment with 160 mg of regorafenib daily on days 1 to 21 every 28 days.

- Of the 901 patients treated, the majority were male (58%), with liver metastases (57%) and *RAS* mutations (59%); they were treated with a median of 2 prior therapies, mainly VEGF-targeted therapy (in 81%).
- 36% of patients had rectal primaries, and 41% had left-sided primary colonic cancers.
- The primary end point of overall survival was significantly better with ZA than with regorafenib (median, 10.9 vs. 9.4 months; hazard ratio, 0.80), with improved survival at 12 months (46% vs. 38%) and 24 months (20% vs. 10%).

- Objective response rates were limited with both ZA (4%) and regorafenib (1%), but disease control was more common with ZA (54% vs. 41%). Progression-free survival was longer with ZA than with regorafenib (median, 3.7 months vs. 2.0 months).
- Treatment-related grade 3 or 4 serious adverse events were more common with ZA than with regorafenib (60% vs. 37%), including hypertension, proteinuria, fatigue, and diarrhea, but no new safety signals emerged.

STELLAR-303 is the first phase 3 randomized trial to demonstrate a survival benefit for an immunotherapy regimen in chemotherapy-refractory metastatic colorectal cancer. If these results lead to FDA approval, this regimen may emerge as a new therapeutic option in chemotherapy-refractory colorectal cancer.

Is Fecal Immunohistochemical Testing (FIT) an Alternative to Colonoscopy in Patients at High Risk for Colon Cancer[117]

A systematic review shows that evidence is inadequate to support FIT testing in such patients.

Patients often are reluctant to undergo colonoscopy for colorectal cancer (CRC) screening. For patients at average risk, stool-based tests are an alternative, but these tests currently are not recommended for patients at higher risk (for example, those with a personal history of polyps or family history of CRC). Researchers performed a systematic review to assess performance of fecal immunohistochemical testing (FIT) in higher-risk populations.

The 14 included studies had heterogeneous designs and used different diagnostic thresholds to define a "positive" FIT test, so variability in reported outcomes was considerable.

In patients with personal history of polyps or family history of CRC, the reported sensitivity of one-time FIT testing to detect CRC ranged from ≈25% to 100%.

A Relatively New Colonoscopic Approach to Large Dysplastic Lesions[119]

In expert hands, endoscopic submucosal dissection achieved complete resection in most cases.

Sometimes a high-risk neoplastic colorectal lesion is not removed completely with standard colonoscopic techniques. A specialized procedure called endoscopic submucosal dissection (ESD) is being used increasingly to resect residual neoplastic tissue during subsequent colonoscopy. In this retrospective study, physicians with expertise in ESD described their experience in 415 cases drawn from a large group of referral centers.

The median size of the colorectal lesion that had been resected incompletely during previous colonoscopy was 3.5 cm; most lesions were adenomas with dysplasia. Outcomes of subsequent ESD were as follows:

- Complete endoscopic resection was achieved in 98% of cases.
- Almost three quarters of resections were considered to be curative, according to prespecified histologic criteria indicating low probability of invasive behavior.
- Intraprocedural perforation occurred in 19 patients: 2 required surgery, and the others were managed endoscopically.
- Three patients had substantial intraprocedural bleeding; all cases were managed endoscopically.
- Delayed postprocedural adverse events occurred in 25 patients, but only 2 of these events (stricture and rectovaginal fistula) required surgery.

General internists and family physicians increasingly might see ESD proposed as a secondary “salvage” procedure in patients with dysplastic but incompletely resected colorectal lesions. This report provides an overview of outcomes and complications, but these outcomes reflect experience from mostly large, well-known referral centers.

Nonoperative Management of Mismatch Repair–Deficient Tumors[130]

Among patients with mismatch repair–deficient (dMMR), locally advanced rectal cancer, neoadjuvant checkpoint blockade eliminated the need for surgery in a high proportion of patients. Whether this approach can be extended to all early-stage dMMR solid tumors, regardless of tumor site, is unknown.

The investigators conducted a phase 2 study in which patients with stage I, II, or III dMMR solid tumors that were amenable to curative-intent surgery were treated with neoadjuvant dostarlimab, a programmed cell death 1 (PD-1) blocking agent, for 6 months. The response to treatment was assessed in two cohorts: patients in cohort 1 had dMMR, locally advanced rectal cancer, and patients in cohort 2 had dMMR nonrectal solid tumors. Patients with a clinical complete response could elect to proceed with nonoperative management; those with residual disease were to undergo resection. In this analysis, the primary end point, assessed in cohort 1, was a sustained clinical complete response at 12 months. Recurrence-free survival and safety were evaluated.

A total of 117 patients were included in the analysis. In cohort 1, all 49 patients who completed treatment had a clinical complete response and elected to proceed with nonoperative management. A total of 37 patients had a sustained clinical complete response at 12 months, a finding that met the criterion for efficacy. In cohort 2, a total of 35 of 54 patients who completed treatment had a clinical complete response, and 33 elected to proceed with nonoperative management. Among the 103 patients who completed treatment across both cohorts, 84 had a clinical complete response, and 82 did not undergo surgery. Among the 117 total patients, recurrence-free survival at 2 years was 92% (95% confidence interval, 86 to 99); the median follow-up for recurrence was 20.0 months (range, 0 to 60.8). The majority of patients (95%) had reversible, grade 1 or 2 adverse events (60%) or had no adverse events (35%). The option for curative resection was not compromised during or after treatment in any of the patients

Among patients with early-stage dMMR solid tumors that were amenable to curative-intent surgery, neoadjuvant PD-1 blockade led to organ preservation in a high proportion of patients.

Combination or Single-Agent Immune Checkpoint Inhibition in MSI-High/dMMR Metastatic Colorectal Cancer?[146]

Progression-free survival and response rate were superior with the combination of ipilimumab and nivolumab compared with nivolumab alone.

For patients with microsatellite instability (MSI)-high/mismatch repair protein-deficient (dMMR) metastatic colorectal cancer, first-line treatment with the immune checkpoint inhibitors pembrolizumab or nivolumab is superior to chemotherapy. The role of dual-targeted versus single-agent immune checkpoint inhibition in these patients, however, remained an unanswered question.

Investigators reported results of the industry-sponsored, open-label, randomized CheckMate 8HW trial comparing single-agent nivolumab with the combination of ipilimumab and nivolumab. The primary endpoint was progression-free survival (PFS) in patients who had centrally confirmed dMMR/MSI-high metastatic colorectal cancer and were being treated in first or later lines of therapy. Of the 707 patients, 57% had received no prior therapy, 68% had right-sided primary cancers, 14% had confirmed Lynch syndrome, and 82% had central confirmation of MSI-high/dMMR status.

At a median follow-up of 47 months, median PFS was superior with ipilimumab/nivolumab compared with single-agent nivolumab (not reached vs. 39.3 months; hazard ratio, 0.62; P=0.0003). At 36 months, 68% of patients in the combination-therapy arm were free of progression compared with 51% of those in the single-agent nivolumab arm. The response rate was significantly higher with combination therapy than with single-agent nivolumab (71% vs. 58%). No new safety signals were observed.

The combination of ipilimumab and nivolumab achieved superior PFS and response compared with single-agent nivolumab and represents a new and arguably preferred standard of care in the first-line treatment of MSH-high/dMMR metastatic colorectal cancer. Overall survival results are pending.

4. ANAL CANCER

First-Line Retifanlimab for Anal Cancer[75]

In patients with advanced anal cancer, superior progression-free survival and responses were achieved with the anti-PD-1 agent retifanlimab.

Standard first-line chemotherapy for patients with advanced anal cancer combines carboplatin and paclitaxel. Immune checkpoint inhibitors have been endorsed for later-line therapy based on modest activity in phase 2 trials. Now, investigators reported results of a global, placebo-controlled, randomized phase 3 trial of the anti-PD-1 agent retifanlimab plus carboplatin and paclitaxel in patients with advanced or metastatic anal squamous cell cancer. Among 308 participants, 72% were female, 70% had received prior radiotherapy, and 91% tested PD-L1–positive at 1% or higher.

Progression-free survival (the primary endpoint) was superior for the addition of retifanlimab versus placebo (9.3 vs. 7.4 months, HR 0.63). Preliminary analysis of median overall survival indicated a trend toward superiority of retifanlimab (29 vs. 23 months). Antitumor responses increased from 44% to 56% with retifanlimab. Incidence of serious treatment-related adverse events was greater with retifanlimab (16% vs 7%).

These practice-changing findings confirm that retifanlimab should be added to first-line chemotherapy in the management of advanced or recurrent anal cancer.

5. PROSTATE CANCER

Is There a Role for Prostate Radiotherapy in De Novo Metastatic Prostate Cancer?[16]

A radiographic progression-free survival benefit was demonstrated in patients with low-volume disease receiving androgen deprivation therapy with intensification.

Overwhelming level 1 evidence supports the addition of androgen receptor pathway inhibitors with or without docetaxel in patients with de novo metastatic castration-sensitive prostate cancer (mCSPC). A meta-analysis of two randomized trials showed evidence of survival benefit from the addition of prostate radiotherapy in men with low-volume metastatic disease (Eur Urol 2019; 76:115).

In this study investigators from the randomized, phase 3 PEACE-1 trial reported the efficacy and safety associated with the addition of prostate radiotherapy to androgen deprivation therapy (ADT), docetaxel, and abiraterone in these patients. In the ongoing open-label trial, 1172 patients with de novo mCSPC were randomly assigned to receive standard of care (ADT) alone, standard of care plus radiotherapy, standard of care plus abiraterone, or standard of care plus abiraterone plus radiotherapy. The trial was later amended to include docetaxel as part of standard of care. Coprimary endpoints were radiographic progression-free survival (rPFS) and overall survival (OS).

At a median follow-up of 6 years, key outcomes were as follows:

1. No OS benefit from the addition of radiotherapy was seen either in the cohort of patients with low-volume disease (<3 bone metastases, no visceral metastases) or in the overall study population.
2. Among patients with low-volume disease, rPFS was significantly improved with the addition of radiotherapy to ADT plus abiraterone, with or without docetaxel.
3. Risk for serious genitourinary adverse events was reduced with radiotherapy both in patients with low-volume disease and in the overall cohort.

Although a previous trial demonstrated an OS benefit from the addition of prostate radiotherapy, that trial did not include patients receiving standard ADT intensification (Lancet 2018; 392:2353). The results from PEACE-1, while not demonstrating an improvement in OS, are compelling enough to consider this option for patients with de novo low-volume metastatic disease managed with ADT intensification using androgen receptor pathway inhibitors.

Diabetes and Heart Disease in Men Who Receive Androgen-Deprivation Therapy[64]

The dramatic increase in the use of androgen-deprivation therapy (primarily in patients with high-PSA-only disease) in the USA during the past decade remains unsupported by prospective evidence of benefit. There is now compelling data showing that androgen-deprivation therapy is associated with higher risk for diabetes, heart disease, and osteoporosis. The reported differences in risk associated with GnRH therapy and orchiectomy require further evaluation.

Since the introduction of prostate-specific antigen (PSA) measurement into clinical practice in the late 1980s, managing patients with prostate cancer has changed dramatically. Use of androgen-deprivation therapy (in many instances, for patients with rising PSA levels only) has increased substantially. Patients with disease identified only by high PSA levels have substantially longer survival than do patients with overt metastatic disease, which results in prolonged exposure to this therapy. Moreover, additional problems, such as treatment-related osteoporosis, now are recognized.

U.S. researchers conducted an observational study of a population-based cohort of 73,196 Medicare enrollees (age, ≥66; mean age, 74) with loco-regional prostate cancer that was diagnosed from 1992 through 1999; patients were observed until 2001. The investigators used a Cox proportional hazards model to assess whether androgen-deprivation therapy was associated with diabetes, coronary artery disease, myocardial infarction, or sudden death.

Overall, 36.3% of patients received a gonadotropin-releasing hormone (GnRH) agonist, and 6.9% underwent bilateral orchiectomy during follow-up. Compared with no hormone use, GnRH-agonist use was significantly associated with increased risk for diabetes, coronary heart disease, and sudden cardiac death. Compared with men who did not receive hormone treatment or undergo surgery, those who underwent orchiectomy were at significantly higher risk for developing diabetes. In adjusted analyses in which the association between disease and duration of GnRH-agonist use was examined, risk for both diabetes and coronary heart disease was higher among men who received therapy for as few as 1 to 4 months than among those who received no GnRH therapy.

Augmenting Androgen Inhibition in Metastatic Castration-Sensitive Prostate Cancer[104]

Patients with HRR mutations had improved radiographic progression-free survival with the addition of a PARP inhibitor to standard of care.

In men with metastatic castration-resistant prostate cancer harboring homologous recombination repair (HRR) gene alterations such as BRCA1 and BRCA2, use of poly(ADP-ribose) polymerase (PARP) inhibitors combined with androgen-receptor pathway inhibitors (ARPI) demonstrates meaningful clinical activity. In this study the investigators asked if a PARP/ARPI combination could also prove effective in men with metastatic castration-sensitive prostate cancer (mCSPC) with HRR mutations. They randomized 700 patients (about half with BRCA1 or BRCA2 mutations) to receive abiraterone acetate and prednisone (AAP) plus either the PARP inhibitor niraparib or placebo. The median follow-up was 2.5 years.

- Treatment with niraparib and AAP significantly improved the primary endpoint of radiographic progression-free survival compared with AAP alone in all patients with HRR mutations (hazard ratio, 0.63; median not reached vs. 30 months) and in the BRCA subgroup (HR, 0.52; median not reached vs. 26 months).
- Overall survival data were immature.
- More patients receiving niraparib/AAP had grade 3 or 4 adverse events (75% vs. 59% with AAP alone).

This is the first phase 3 trial to demonstrate efficacy of a PARP inhibitor in mCSPC, but some caution is required. Data on overall survival remain immature, and the higher rate of severe adverse events with niraparib is a concern.

Variability in PSA Levels During Prostate Cancer Screening[106]

Men with at least one PSA level ≥4.0 ng/mL often had subsequent levels below that threshold.

The American Urological Association (AUA) recommends that men with elevated prostate-specific antigen (PSA) levels on screening undergo repeat testing “a few months” later, before being referred to a urologist for further evaluation. This recommendation reflects the fact that PSA levels can fluctuate over relatively short to intermediate timeframes.

In this study, researchers examined how often PSA levels above commonly used thresholds (4.0 and 3.0 ng/mL) drop to below those thresholds by the next annual screening. They used data from 11,000 men in the PLCO screening trial (age range, 54–75) who were screened annually for up to 6 years and were not diagnosed with prostate cancer during the trial.

PSA levels at or above 4.0 ng/mL fell below that threshold on the next annual test 30% of the time.

Roughly 60% of patients had at least one instance where their PSA level was ≥4.0 ng/mL and then dropped below that threshold on the next annual test.

Similar results were seen with a threshold of 3.0 ng/mL.

PSA is a problematic screening test: There is no threshold level above which the incidence of clinically important prostate cancer changes dramatically. This study was not designed to settle the question of what threshold is optimal to maximize benefit and minimize downstream harms from overdiagnosis. However, it does quantitate what is often seen in clinical practice, and it supports the AUA recommendation that patients undergo repeat testing before being referred for possible biopsy.

Long-Term Outcomes from a Landmark Prostate Cancer Screening Trial[116]

Screening was associated with 22 fewer prostate cancer deaths per 10,000 men.

The European Randomized Study of Screening for Prostate Cancer, with 182,000 participants, is considered the most credible of several randomized trials of prostate-specific antigen (PSA) screening for prostate cancer. Initial findings, published in 2009 after 9 years of follow-up, indicated seven fewer prostate cancer deaths per 10,000 screened men compared with controls. Now, the researchers have provided longer-term outcomes.

At 23 years, cumulative prostate cancer mortality was 1.4% in the screening group and 1.6% in the control group, a statistically significant difference that translates into 22 fewer prostate cancer deaths per 10,000 men. As expected in a screening study, prostate cancer was diagnosed significantly more frequently in the screening group than in the control group (14% vs. 12%).

Further improvement in prostate cancer–specific mortality with extended follow-up of the European Randomized Study of Screening for Prostate Cancer participants is reassuring. Moreover, in contemporary practice, greater use of magnetic resonance imaging and of surveillance in patients with low-grade cancers has refined our decision-making in men with elevated PSA levels.

Improved Survival with Enzalutamide in Biochemically Recurrent Prostate Cancer[124]

In the phase 3 EMBARK trial, enzalutamide plus leuprolide and enzalutamide monotherapy were associated with longer metastasis-free survival than leuprolide alone among patients with biochemically recurrent prostate cancer. The final analysis of overall survival has not been previously reported. Overall survival was significantly longer with the combination of enzalutamide and leuprolide than with leuprolide alone among patients with prostate cancer with high-risk biochemical recurrence. Enzalutamide monotherapy was not superior to leuprolide alone in the analysis of overall survival.

The investigators randomly assigned patients with prostate cancer who had high-risk biochemical recurrence in a 1:1:1 ratio to receive enzalutamide plus leuprolide (the combination group), leuprolide alone (the leuprolide-alone group), or enzalutamide monotherapy (the monotherapy group). The primary end point was metastasis-free survival, assessed in the combination group as compared with the leuprolide-alone group. Updated results for prespecified secondary end points, including the time to first use of new antineoplastic therapy and the time to the first symptomatic skeletal event, were summarized descriptively, as was progression-free survival with the first subsequent therapy.

The 8-year overall survival was 78.9% (95% confidence interval [CI], 73.9 to 83.1) in the combination group and 69.5% (95% CI, 64.0 to 74.3) in the leuprolide-alone group; the hazard ratio for death was 0.60 (95% CI, 0.44 to 0.80; P<0.001). The 8-year overall survival with monotherapy was 73.1% (95% CI, 67.6 to 77.9), which did not differ significantly from that with leuprolide alone (hazard ratio, 0.83; 95% CI, 0.63 to 1.10; P=0.19). In the descriptive updates for prespecified secondary end points, results were similar to those previously reported. Safety findings were consistent with those in the primary analysis of metastasis-free survival.

When Is Prostate Cancer Really Cancer?[145]

Experts in the field debated whether Gleason 6 prostate neoplasia should be labeled as "cancer."

A group of 50 experts in prostate cancer, representing numerous specialty areas, met recently to address whether low-grade prostate neoplasia (Gleason 6 or Grade Group 1 [GG1]) should be called "cancer". The participants did not come to final conclusions, but their deliberations, including 36 commissioned presentations and discussions, should interest both specialists and primary care clinicians.

Prostate cancer is graded histologically by pathologists on a scale of 1 to 5 (from no to highly cancerous features). The scores of the primary histologic pattern and the most common secondary pattern are added together. Prostate cancer is not diagnosed when this score is ≤5, so the range of scores for a lesion labeled as "cancer" is 6 to 10. A Gleason score of 6 (i.e., 3+3) is termed GG1.

In autopsy series, GG1 lesions are so ubiquitous that many experts believe them to be a normal feature of aging. Pure GG1 lesions cause no symptoms, and, if they don't change during follow-up, they remain asymptomatic and do not metastasize. Overtreatment of persistent, but unchanging, GG1 lesions causes substantial and avoidable morbidity, without improving all-cause or cancer-specific mortality. However, GG1 lesions should not be considered "normal" by physicians nor presented as such to patients. Because they potentially can progress to more-aggressive, clinically significant disease, active surveillance should be offered. Summit participants speculated that a commitment to active surveillance by both physician and patient might be more productively discussed if GG1 lesions are renamed and not called "cancer."

The authors also argued that enthusiasm and support among clinicians for early screening, including prostate-specific antigen (PSA) testing, might improve if a clear consensus is reached about how to discuss and manage GG1 lesions. Although a majority of GG1 cases in the U.S.A. now are managed with active surveillance, local variation in practice still occurs. According to the authors, "GG1 should nearly always be managed with initial active surveillance or observation." A marked reduction in immediate treatment of GG1 might improve patients' acceptance of more-regular screening, leading to earlier detection of aggressive lesions.

Two concerns about a name change were expressed. First, adherence to an active-surveillance program might be low if the lesion is not labeled as "cancer." And second, active surveillance or more-aggressive management of patients at high risk (including those with early and strong family history of cancer) might not be supported by health insurance plans if the lesion is not labeled as "cancer."

One proposed name for GG1 lesions is "acinar neoplasm." The renaming process could benefit from the experience of thyroid cancer experts who worked through a process of renaming one indolent variant of papillary thyroid neoplasia — previously labeled as “cancer” — to “noninvasive follicular thyroid neoplasm with papillary-like nuclear features.”

In summary, this conference of expert opinion opened a critical discussion about how to name a histological abnormality of the prostate. Patients with GG1 lesions are generally managed by urologists, but primary care clinicians are often asked by patients for their opinion about treatment alternatives and should be informed about this debate and be prepared to engage in shared decision making if requested. Similar discussions are underway regarding how to name and manage ductal carcinoma in situ (DCIS) of the breast, but that field is less developed because long-term DCIS data are scant compared with that of GG1 prostate lesions

6. BLADDER CANCER/UROTHELIAL CARCINOMA

Adjuvant Pembrolizumab versus Observation in Muscle-Invasive Urothelial Carcinoma[24]

Among patients with high-risk muscle-invasive urothelial carcinoma after radical surgery, disease-free survival was significantly longer with adjuvant pembrolizumab than with observation.

In this phase 3 trial, the investigators randomly assigned patients, in a 1:1 ratio, to receive pembrolizumab at a dose of 200 mg every 3 weeks for 1 year or to undergo observation. Randomization was stratified according to pathological stage, centrally tested programmed death ligand 1 (PD-L1) status, and previous neoadjuvant chemotherapy. The coprimary end points were disease-free survival and overall survival in the intention-to-treat population.

A total of 702 patients underwent randomization; 354 were assigned to receive pembrolizumab, and 348 were assigned to observation. As of July 5, 2024, the median duration of follow-up for disease-free survival was 44.8 months. The median disease-free survival was 29.6 months (95% confidence interval [CI], 20.0 to 40.7) with pembrolizumab and 14.2 months (95% CI, 11.0 to 20.2) with observation (hazard ratio for disease progression or death, 0.73; 95% CI, 0.59 to 0.90; two-sided P=0.003). Grade 3 or higher adverse events (regardless of attribution) occurred in

50.6% of the patients in the pembrolizumab group and in 31.6% of the patients in the observation group.

ctDNA-Guided Adjuvant Atezolizumab in Muscle-Invasive Bladder Cancer[122]

Among patients with muscle-invasive bladder cancer, ctDNA-guided adjuvant therapy with atezolizumab led to significantly longer disease-free survival and overall survival than placebo.

Patients with muscle-invasive bladder cancer have varied outcomes after cystectomy. Circulating tumor DNA (ctDNA)–based detection of molecular residual disease may identify patients at high risk for recurrence after cystectomy who can benefit from adjuvant immunotherapy, thus sparing patients at lower risk from unnecessary treatment burden.

In a phase 3, double-blind, randomized trial, the investigators used serial ctDNA testing to monitor (for up to 1 year) patients with muscle-invasive bladder cancer and no radiographic evidence of disease after surgery. Eligible patients who tested ctDNA-positive during surveillance were randomly assigned in a 2:1 ratio to receive intravenous atezolizumab or placebo every 4 weeks for up to 1 year. The primary end point was investigator-assessed disease-free survival. Overall survival was a secondary end point that was assessed in a hierarchical fashion to control for alpha. Patients who persistently tested ctDNA-negative did not receive atezolizumab or placebo.

A total of 761 patients were enrolled; 250 eligible patients who tested ctDNA-positive underwent randomization (167 to the atezolizumab group and 83 to the placebo group). The median disease-free survival was 9.9 months with atezolizumab, as compared with 4.8 months with placebo (hazard ratio for first event of disease recurrence or death, 0.64; 95% confidence interval [CI], 0.47 to 0.87; P=0.005). The median overall survival was 32.8 months with atezolizumab, as compared with 21.1 months with placebo (hazard ratio for death, 0.59; 95% CI, 0.39 to 0.90; P=0.01). A total of 28% of the patients who received atezolizumab and 22% of those who received placebo had adverse events of grade 3 or 4 (related to atezolizumab or placebo in 7% vs. 4%); 3% and 2% of the patients, respectively, had fatal adverse events (related to atezolizumab or placebo in 2% vs. none). Among 357 patients with persistent ctDNA-negative status, disease-free survival was 95% at the end of the 1-year monitoring period and 88% at 2 years.

Among patients with muscle-invasive bladder cancer, ctDNA-guided adjuvant therapy with atezolizumab led to significantly longer disease-free survival and overall survival than placebo.

Disitamab Vedotin plus Toripalimab in HER2-Expressing Advanced Urothelial Cancer[123]

Disitamab vedotin–toripalimab led to a significantly greater improvement in outcomes than chemotherapy among patients with untreated HER2-expressing locally advanced or metastatic urothelial cancer.

Human epidermal growth factor receptor 2 (HER2)–directed antibody–drug conjugate monotherapy has shown preliminary clinical efficacy in patients with chemotherapy-refractory HER2-positive locally advanced or metastatic urothelial cancer. Previous data showed promising antitumor activity and safety of HER2-specific disitamab vedotin as monotherapy and when combined with programmed cell death protein 1 (PD-1)–directed immunotherapy in this cancer.

In this phase 3, multicenter, open-label, randomized trial, the investigators assigned patients with previously untreated HER2-expressing (immunohistochemical score of 1+, 2+, or 3+) locally advanced or metastatic urothelial cancer in a 1:1 ratio to receive either disitamab vedotin plus PD-1–specific toripalimab every 2 weeks or chemotherapy (gemcitabine plus cisplatin or carboplatin) every 3 weeks. The dual primary end points were progression-free survival (assessed by blinded independent review) and overall survival. Secondary end points included objective response and safety. The prespecified progression-free survival analysis and interim overall survival analysis are presented in this paper.

A total of 484 patients underwent randomization. The median follow-up was 18.2 months. Progression-free survival was significantly longer in the disitamab vedotin–toripalimab group than in the chemotherapy group (median, 13.1 vs. 6.5 months; hazard ratio for progression or death, 0.36; 95% confidence interval [CI], 0.28 to 0.46; P<0.001). Overall survival was also significantly longer in the disitamab vedotin–toripalimab group than in the chemotherapy group (median, 31.5 vs. 16.9 months; hazard ratio for death, 0.54; 95% CI, 0.41 to 0.73; P<0.001). The

percentage of patients with an objective response was 76.1% (95% CI, 70.3 to 81.3) in the disitamab vedotin–toripalimab group and 50.2% (95% CI, 43.7 to 56.7) in the chemotherapy group. The safety profile of disitamab vedotin plus toripalimab was more favorable than that of chemotherapy; grade 3 or higher treatment-related adverse events occurred in 55.1% of patients who received disitamab vedotin plus toripalimab and 86.9% of those who received chemotherapy.
Disitamab vedotin–toripalimab led to a significantly greater improvement in outcomes than chemotherapy among patients with untreated HER2-expressing locally advanced or metastatic urothelial cancer.

7. RENAL CANCER

Is an Effective Treatment for Hereditary and Sporadic Papillary Kidney Cancer at Hand?[87]

Two wellknown therapeutic agents, when combined, were effective in this rare disease subset.

Hereditary leiomyomatosis and renal cell cancer (HLRCC) is a hereditary condition caused by germline mutations in the fumarate hydratase gene, which increase the risk for an aggressive papillary renal cell cancer that lacks effective therapy. In preclinical studies using HLRCC models, blockade of both vascular endothelial growth factor (VEGF) receptor and epidermal growth factor receptor (EGFR) provided significant antitumor activity. Now, investigators have conducted an open-label, phase II trial of the combination of the VEGFA blocker bevacizumab and the EGFR blocker erlotinib in 40 patients with sporadic papillary renal cell carcinoma and 43 patients with HLRCC-associated papillary renal cell carcinoma. The primary end point was overall response rate.

Patients with HLRCC had a median age of 43 years compared with 56 years in the sporadic arm. Approximately one third of all patients had received at least one prior line of therapy. During a median follow-up of 72 months in the HLRCC group and 64 months in the sporadic-carcinoma group, the overall response rate was 72% (including 2 with complete response) in the HLRCC group and 35% in the sporadic-carcinoma group. In the HLRCC group, the median progression-free survival was 21.1 months, 15 patients continued therapy for more than 2 years, and the median overall survival was 44.6 months. Adverse events were consistent with the side effect profile of these two agents: Rash, diarrhea, and proteinuria were most common.

When managing patients with rare renal cancer histology, clinicians typically extrapolate therapeutic approaches from large studies in patients with clear cell renal cancer or smaller phase II trials in non–clear cell subtypes. This study provides a viable therapeutic alternative for this rare renal cancer subgroup

Is Renal Ultrasound a Viable Approach for Evaluating Microhematuria?[118]

Among 5000 patients with microhematuria, 5 kidney cancers and 1 bladder cancer identified by CT or MRI were missed by concurrent renal ultrasound.

Recent guidelines from the American Urological Association published in 2020 and amended in 2025) recommend renal ultrasound rather than cross-sectional imaging (i.e., computed tomography or magnetic resonance imaging [CT/MRI]) for evaluating patients with microhematuria who are at low or intermediate risk. In this study, researchers in Texas used a large, single-institution database to assess the diagnostic efficiency of this approach in more than 5000 outpatients (mean age, 52) with microhematuria, defined as ≥3 red blood cells per high-power field. About half of patients were classified as having low or intermediate risk based on age, sex, and smoking status. Patients with prior genitourinary malignancy were excluded.

Cancers were identified in 47 patients (0.91%) by one or more forms of imaging (32 renal, 12 bladder, and 3 upper-tract urothelial carcinoma). Among 401 patients with initial negative renal ultrasound, 5 cancers were diagnosed by subsequent CT/MRI within 3 months. All 5 patients had renal cancer, and 3 patients were at high risk.

Of 12 bladder cancers diagnosed by imaging, 10 were diagnosed initially by CT and 2 were diagnosed by renal ultrasound. Only 1 of the CT-identified cancers was missed by renal ultrasound (and that patient was at high risk). Only 1 bladder cancer was diagnosed by cystoscopy and missed on CT.

These results confirmed the American Urological Association's recommendation to use renal ultrasound in initial evaluation of patients with microscopic hematuria who are at low or intermediate risk.

8. HEAD AND NECK CANCER

Cetuximab plus Postoperative Radiotherapy for Intermediate Risk Head and Neck Cancer?[45]

The addition of cetuximab to postoperative radiotherapy improved disease-free survival but did not confer an overall survival benefit and was associated with increased toxicity.

Postoperative chemoradiation with cisplatin is the standard of care for locally advanced head and neck squamous cell carcinoma (HNSCC) in patients with high risk for recurrence (e.g., pathologic findings of positive margins, extranodal extension of tumor). Whether patients with intermediate-risk disease would benefit from concurrent systemic therapy with postoperative radiation is unclear.

This multicenter, open-label, randomized phase 3 trial evaluated the efficacy of adding cetuximab to postoperative radiotherapy (RT) in patients with resected intermediate-risk HNSCC (close [<5 mm] resection margins, pathologic stage T3 or T4a tumors, pathologic N2 disease, lymphovascular or perineural invasion, or T2 oral cavity cancer with >5mm depth of invasion).

Of 577 patients randomized to RT alone or RT plus cetuximab, 18% had HPV-positive oropharynx cancer, and the majority had HPV-negative oral cavity (63.6%) or larynx (14.2%) cancers. At a median follow-up of 7.2 years, the addition of cetuximab to postoperative RT did not significantly improve overall survival (the primary endpoint) compared with RT alone (hazard ratio, 0.81; P=0.08) but did significantly improve disease-free survival (HR, 0.75; P=0.02). Cetuximab was associated with more grade 3–4 adverse events than RT alone (70.3% vs. 39.7%), particularly lymphopenia and dermatologic and infusion-related events.

Cetuximab was previously shown to be inferior to cisplatin when given with definitive radiation in HPV-positive, locally advanced HNSCC, with comparable toxicity (Lancet 2019; 393:40). The current study suggests that while cetuximab may delay disease recurrence, it does not improve long-term survival and carries added toxicity. Of note, subgroup analyses suggested that HPV-negative tumors and tumors with 3 or more risk features are more likely to benefit from the addition of cetuximab.

However, the trial highlights the need for further research to refine risk stratification and identify optimal adjuvant therapies for intermediate-risk HNSCC.

Can Perioperative Pembrolizumab Improve Outcomes in Locally Advanced Head and Neck Cancer?[71]

Yes: the KEYNOTE-689 trial showed a significant event-free survival improvement.

Immune checkpoint inhibitors (ICIs) have established roles in recurrent and metastatic squamous cell carcinoma of the head and neck (HNSCC), whereas ICIs combined with definitive chemoradiation failed to improve outcomes in the curative-intent, locally advanced setting. To explore a role for perioperative administration of ICIs, investigators randomized more than 700 patients newly diagnosed with resectable locally advanced HNSCC to receive standard-of-care treatment (surgery plus adjuvant radiotherapy with or without cisplatin) either alone or with perioperative pembrolizumab (2 cycles neoadjuvant followed by 15 cycles adjuvant starting with radiation). Results of the multicenter, phase 3 KEYNOTE-689 trial were as follows:

Patients who received pembrolizumab maintained longer event-free survival (EFS) at 3 years than those who did not (58% vs. 46%; hazard ratio, 0.73). Overall survival trended favorably (68% vs. 61% at 3 years; HR, 0.76).

All patients benefited regardless of PD-L1 expression levels, but those whose percentage of tumor cells and immune cells containing PD-L1 was ≥10 appeared to benefit the most (3-year EFS, 60% vs. 46% HR, 0.66). More patients in the pembrolizumab group than the control group had a major pathological response (9% vs. none).

Adverse events were manageable and consistent with the known pembrolizumab safety profile, although immune-related adverse events occurred more frequently with pembrolizumab.

These positive results with perioperative pembrolizumab contrast with previous ICI studies in nonsurgical settings. Additional mature survival data will further define the role of ICIs in this setting.

Does Neoadjuvant/Induction Chemotherapy Benefit High-Risk, Locally Advanced Nasopharyngeal Carcinoma?[140]

Adding four cycles of neoadjuvant docetaxel and cisplatin before definitive chemoradiotherapy significantly improved distant metastasis–free and overall survival in patients with N2–3 disease.

Nasopharyngeal carcinoma (NPC) is a unique subset of head and neck cancers strongly associated with Epstein-Barr virus infection and prone to distant metastasis. While concurrent chemoradiotherapy (CRT), with or without induction and/or adjuvant systemic therapy, is the standard of care for locoregionally advanced NPC, patients with extensive nodal involvement (N2–3) remain at high risk for systemic failure.

In this multicenter, open-label, phase 3 trial conducted in China, 186 patients with newly diagnosed stage T1–4, N2–3, M0 NPC were randomized to receive either four cycles of neoadjuvant docetaxel (75 mg/m^2 on day 1) and cisplatin (37.5 mg/m^2 on days 2–3) followed by CRT, or CRT alone.

At a median follow-up of 76.9 months, the addition of neoadjuvant chemotherapy significantly improved 5-year distant metastasis–free survival (91.3% vs. 78.2%; hazard ratio, 0.41) and overall survival (90.3% vs. 82.6%; HR, 0.38). Grade 3–4 acute toxicities were more common in the neoadjuvant group (65% vs. 51%), mainly due to neutropenia (47% vs. 11%), but no differences in late toxicities or long-term quality of life were observed.

This is the first phase 3 trial focused exclusively on N2–3 NPC. By targeting N2–3 disease, the study enriched for patients most likely to benefit from intensified systemic therapy. Immunotherapy-based approaches, although promising, are often costlier, less accessible, and associated with immune-related toxicities. This trial demonstrates that a cytotoxic regimen using docetaxel and cisplatin — a widely available and relatively cost-effective option — can deliver substantial benefit when used selectively in high-risk patients and highlights the importance of risk-adapted strategies in NPC management, particularly in resource-constrained settings. This treatment also could be an option for patients who are not fit for a higher cisplatin bolus (75 mg/m^2) with gemcitabine and cisplatin induction.

Can Adjuvant Atezolizumab Improve Outcomes in Locally Advanced Squamous Cell Carcinoma of the Head and Neck?[142]

A third trial demonstrated no benefit from adding an immune checkpoint inhibitor to definitive multimodality therapy in this setting.

Immune checkpoint inhibitors (ICIs) have been shown to improve survival in patients with recurrent and/or metastatic squamous cell carcinoma of the head and neck (SCCHN), but their use in locally advanced SCCHN has been less successful. Two previous clinical trials evaluating the addition of ICIs to concurrent definitive chemoradiation failed to demonstrate improvements in progression-free or event-free survival (EFS) Now, investigators have reported results from a study of adjuvant ICI therapy.

In this multinational, phase 3 trial, 406 patients who had undergone multimodal definitive treatment for high-risk locally advanced SCCHN were randomized to receive either atezolizumab (1200 mg) or placebo every 3 weeks for up to 1 year. Approximately 62% of patients had received primary nonsurgical management (chemoradiation or induction chemotherapy followed by radiation or chemoradiation); the remainder had received surgery followed by radiation or chemoradiation, or induction chemotherapy followed by surgery with or without radiation.

At a median follow-up of 46.5 months, the median EFS (the primary endpoint) was not significantly different between the atezolizumab and placebo groups (59.5 and 52.7 months); this finding was consistent across subgroups. Overall survival rates at 24 months were also similar (82.0% and 79.2%). Treatment-related adverse events were manageable and consistent with previously known profiles.

This is the third study to show no benefit from adding an ICI to definitive multimodal treatment for locally advanced SCCHN. In contrast, recently announced preliminary results from the GORTEC 2018-01 trial suggest significant improvements in disease-free survival with the use of postoperative nivolumab alongside adjuvant chemoradiation. The Keynote-689 study has also released positive preliminary results demonstrating EFS benefit of neoadjuvant and adjuvant pembrolizumab as perioperative treatment for SCCHN.

Adjuvant Camrelizumab in Locally Advanced Nasopharyngeal Carcinoma[143]

Adding this PD-1 inhibitor after completion of induction chemotherapy and definitive chemoradiation significantly improved event-free survival without negatively affecting quality of life.

Most nasopharyngeal carcinomas (NPCs) express PD-L1, making them excellent targets for PD-1 immunotherapy. In a recent phase 3, randomized trial (CONTINUUM), researchers found that adding the anti–PD-1 antibody sintilimab to induction and concurrent therapies in patients with locally advanced NPC led to significant improvements in event-free survival (EFS). Now, investigators reported on the anti–PD-1 antibody camrelizumab as adjuvant therapy for locoregionally advanced NPC.

In this phase 3, open-label, multicenter trial in China (DIPPER), 450 patients with locoregionally advanced NPC who had already completed induction chemotherapy and definitive chemoradiation were randomized to adjuvant camrelizumab intravenously every 3 weeks for 12 cycles or standard observation. In the primary endpoint analysis, adjuvant camrelizumab significantly improved 3-year EFS compared with observation (86.9% vs. 77.3%; hazard ratio, 0.56). It was also associated with significantly reduced risks of distant metastasis (HR, 0.54) and locoregional relapse (HR, 0.53). Overall survival was similar between the groups at 3 years (96.4% and 92.9%). Reactive capillary endothelial proliferation was the most common adverse event, occurring in 85.8% of patients, but was mostly mild. Grade 3 or 4 adverse events were more common with camrelizumab than with observation (11.2% vs. 3.2%); no significant deterioration in health-related quality of life was observed.

Camrelizumab yielded similar survival benefits to those seen with sintilimab in the CONTINUUM trial but with a much lower rate of grade 3–4 adverse events. This lower rate may be related to camrelizumab being used as adjuvant monotherapy (whereas sintilimab was given from induction therapy onward) or to patient selection in the DIPPER trial: 31% of patients screened were excluded, mostly because of problems during induction or definitive chemoradiation.

Can stereotactic ablative radiation Help Avoid Systemic Therapy in Oligometastatic Squamous Cell Carcinoma of the Head and Neck?[144]

When treated with stereotactic ablative radiation therapy (SABR) alone, patients were spared from toxicities of systemic therapy while achieving similar overall survival to those treated with SABR and systemic chemotherapy.

The standard approach for metastatic squamous cell carcinoma of the head and neck (SCCHN) has been systemic chemotherapy, although it is associated with significant toxicity and quality-of-life (QoL) deterioration. For patients with oligometastatic disease — an intermediate clinical state between locoregional and widely metastatic cancer — targeted therapies such as stereotactic ablative radiation therapy (SABR) may provide prolonged survival with more-acceptable toxicity. In this phase 2 trial (NCT03070366), 69 patients with SCCHN and one to three oligometastases were randomized to either SABR alone or with chemotherapy and immunotherapy (5-fluorouracil, platinum, cetuximab).

The primary endpoint — 1-year overall survival (OS) without QoL deterioration — was similar between the two groups (55.2% and 53.3%). However, patients receiving SABR alone experienced markedly less-severe QoL deterioration and substantially lower rates of grade 3 to 4 adverse events (8.8%, compared with 60.0% with chemo-SABR). Median progression-free survival was numerically shorter with SABR alone (7.4 months) than with chemo-SABR (12.9 months), but OS was similar (41.1 and 42.3 months).

The SABR-alone arm had a slightly higher chance of developing both new metastases and local progression (16.7%) than did the chemo-SABR arm (3.7%), although rate of progression with new metastases only was similar in both arms (50.0% and 55.6%).

This study had several notable limitations: it did not meet its target enrollment, it was conducted before the widespread adoption of immune checkpoint inhibitors, and it failed to achieve its primary objective of at least 50% 1-year OS without QoL deterioration in the SABR-alone arm — although the raw percentage was 55.2%, the lower bound of the confidence interval (0.38) fell below the targeted threshold (0.50). Nonetheless, SABR alone could be useful for carefully selected patients with oligometastatic SCCHN, as it may be a viable alternative to standard chemotherapy with comparable survival outcomes. Importantly, SABR alone considerably preserved patients' quality of life and reduced severe treatment-related toxicities.

9. GASTRIC CARCINOMA AND GASTRO-ESOPHOGEAL CARCINOMA

Early Switch to Paclitaxel/Ramucirumab in Gastric Cancer?[8]

A change to paclitaxel/ramucirumab achieved superior PFS compared with continuation of chemotherapy in patients with disease control after 3 months of initial chemotherapy.

Standard first-line chemotherapy for HER2-negative, PDL1-positive metastatic esophagogastric cancer includes an immune checkpoint inhibitor. Standard chemotherapy at progression is paclitaxel and ramucirumab. Investigators in Italy reported results of an open-label, randomized, phase 3 ARMANI trial comparing continuation of first line FOLFOX or capecitabine/oxaliplatin to an early therapy change to paclitaxel/ramucirumab in 280 patients with metastatic, HER2-negative esophagogastric adenocarcinoma who had achieved disease control (45% stable disease, 41% partial response) after 3 months of initial chemotherapy. No patient received an immune checkpoint inhibitor.

At a median follow-up of 44 months, the primary endpoint of progression-free survival (PFS) was superior for the therapy change compared with continuation (median, 6.6 vs. 3.5 months; hazard ratio, 0.61; P=0.0002). Overall survival (OS) favored therapy change over continuation (12.6 vs. 10.4 months; HR, 0.75; P=0.025). Rates of further response to treatment were similar in the two groups (19% and 16%), with a higher rate of disease control in the therapy change group (85% vs. 54%). Grade 3/4 treatment-related adverse events were more common in the therapy change group (40% vs. 21%). In a post hoc analysis, PFS and OS benefits were limited to patients with stable disease after initial chemotherapy. Only 45% of the continuation group received the standard paclitaxel/ramucirumab at progression. (Ramucirumab is a human vascular endothelial growth factor receptor 2 (VEGFR2) antagonist).

Median PFS with FOLFOX is 6–7 months, so a median PFS of 3.5 months in patients already treated with 3 months of FOLFOX/capecitabine oxaliplatin is not surprising. The PFS results for an early change to paclitaxel/ramucirumab are similar to those reported for this regimen used only at progression.

A Potential New Treatment Option for Chemotherapy-Refractory Gastric Cancer[14]

Regorafenib offers a modest survival benefit over placebo in patients who have received two or more lines of chemotherapy.

For patients with metastatic esophagogastric adenocarcinoma, inhibition of the vascular endothelial growth factor (VEGF) pathway via the anti–VEGFR-2 antibody ramucirumab increases response, progression-free survival (PFS) and overall survival (OS) when combined with second-line treatment with paclitaxel. The multitargeted tyrosine kinase inhibitor regorafenib targets VEGFR and other pathways and has effectiveness in chemotherapy-refractory colorectal cancer.

Investigators now reported results of a randomized, double-blind, placebo-controlled INTEGRATE IIa trial evaluating regorafenib (160 mg daily for 21 days of 28-day cycles) in patients with chemotherapy-refractory esophagogastric adenocarcinoma. Of the 251 patients enrolled, 63% were treated in Asia; 73% had gastric primaries; 42% had received a prior VEGF inhibitor; 59% had received two and 40% had received three or more lines of prior chemotherapy. For the analysis of OS, the primary endpoint, results were pooled with those from INTEGRATE I, a prior randomized, placebo-controlled, phase II trial in 147 patients.

At a median follow-up of 48 months, OS was improved with regorafenib over placebo in the pooled cohort (hazard ratio, 0.70; P=0.001) and in the INTEGRATE IIa cohort (HR, 0.68; P=0.006). In the INTEGRATE IIa cohort, 1-year OS was improved with regorafenib (19% vs. 6%), whereas median OS was similar (4.0 and 4.5 months). PFS was improved with regorafenib (HR, 0.53; P<0.0001). The disease control rate was higher with regorafenib than placebo (21.3% vs. 4.9%) and the antitumor response was limited (2.4% vs. 0%). Adverse events related to regorafenib, including palmar–plantar erythrodysesthesia, mucositis, hypertension, and diarrhea, were manageable.

INTEGRATE IIa indicates a modest improvement in OS and PFS with regorafenib, and limited antitumor responses, in patients with chemotherapy-refractory esophagogastric adenocarcinoma. Regorafenib may emerge as another therapeutic option in these patients, in addition to the recently FDA-approved option of trifluridine tipiracil.

Perioperative Chemotherapy vs. Preoperative Chemoradiotherapy for Resectable Esophageal Carcinoma[21]

Another trial finds no survival benefit from the addition of radiotherapy to preoperative chemotherapy in these patients.

Including radiation therapy in the preoperative treatment of gastroesophageal adenocarcinoma resulted in no survival benefit over chemotherapy alone in two previously reported trials. Investigators in this study reported results of the multicenter, phase 3 ESOPEC trial in which patients with esophageal or gastroesophageal junction (GEJ) adenocarcinoma were randomized to perioperative treatment with FLOT chemotherapy (fluorouracil, leucovorin, oxaliplatin, and docetaxel) or preoperative chemoradiotherapy with carboplatin, paclitaxel, and radiotherapy (41.4 Gy).

Of the 438 patients, 80% had clinical stage T3–4 disease, 80% were node positive, 46% had esophageal or Siewert I GEJ primaries, and 31% had Siewert II GEJ primaries. On the FLOT arm, 89% of patients completed all preoperative chemotherapy and 53% completed all postoperative chemotherapy; on the chemoradiotherapy arm, 89% completed all planned radiotherapy and 68% completed all planned chemotherapy.

The primary endpoint of overall survival was superior with FLOT compared with chemoradiotherapy at 3 years (57.4% vs. 50.7%; hazard ratio, 0.70; *P*=0.01) and at 5 years (50.6% vs. 38.7%). The survival benefit with FLOT was seen across planned subgroups. Progression-free survival at 3 years was also superior with FLOT compared with chemoradiotherapy (51.6% vs. 35.0%; HR, 0.66), as was pathologic complete response (16.7% vs. 10.1%, respectively). No new safety concerns were observed.

This trial showed that FLOT was superior to chemoradiotherapy with carboplatin and paclitaxel, indicating that a superior and more-intensive systemic chemotherapy improved outcome, and that radiation therapy was not required.

Targeting PD-L1 in Gastric Cancer[29]

Adding the anti-PD-L1 antibody sugemalimab to first-line chemotherapy improved survival.

Immune checkpoint inhibitors targeting programmed death protein 1 (PD-1 (edincluding nivolumab, pembrolizumab, and tislelizumab) are combined with first-line chemotherapy in advanced gastric cancer, but the survival benefit is limited to patients testing positive for anti–programmed death-ligand 1 (PD-L1).

Investigators in China report results of a randomized, placebo-controlled GEMSTONE-303 trial evaluating the addition of the anti–PD-L1 agent sugemalimab to first line chemotherapy in patients with advanced gastric cancer and a PD-L1 combined positive score (CPS) >5%. Of the 479 patients treated with capecitabine/oxaliplatin combined with either sugemalimab or placebo, 90% had prior gastrectomy, 39% had hepatic metastases, 46% had CPS scores 5–9%, and 54% had scores >10%.

The co-primary endpoint of overall survival was improved for sugemalimab over placebo (median, 15.6 vs. 12.6 months; hazard ratio, 0.75), as was the coprimary endpoint of progression-free survival (7.6 vs. 6.1 months; HR, 0.66). Response rates were higher with sugemalimab compared with placebo (69% vs. 53%). No new safety signals were observed. Rates of grade 3–5 serious treatment-related adverse events were similar in the sugemalimab and placebo groups (54% and 51%).

Thus, GEMSTONE-303 adds to the list of positive trials evaluating the addition of immune checkpoint inhibitors to first-line chemotherapy in advanced gastric cancer and is the only trial to limit enrollment to patients testing positive for PD-L1 expression. It is also the first trial to validate that an agent targeting PD-L1, not PD-1, improves outcomes when added to first-line chemotherapy.

Preventing Gastric Cancer by Eradicating Helicobacter pylori[68]

A meta-analysis suggested that H. pylori eradication lowers gastric cancer incidence by about 40%.

Gastric infection with Helicobacter pylori initiates mucosal changes that can evolve to adenocarcinoma. Researchers conducted a meta-analysis of 11 randomized trials and 13 cohort studies that compared outcomes in treated and untreated H. pylori–positive adults. In both groups of studies, gastric cancer incidence was 40% lower in people who underwent H. pylori eradication. All but two of these studies were from eastern Asia.

In a retrospective study from Nordic countries (Denmark, Sweden, Norway, Finland, and Iceland), researchers tracked outcomes among 700,000 people treated for H. pylori infection. The incidence of gastric carcinoma was twice that of the general population in the first 5 years after treatment, likely reflecting H. pylori–related carcinogenesis that already was underway, but after 11 years, the incidence fell to that of the general population and remained there.

Together, these two reports provide additional evidence that eradicating H. pylori can lower risk for gastric cancer, not only in Asian countries with a high prevalence of gastric cancer but also in non-Asian populations.

In the U.S., routine screening for gastric cancer or H. pylori infection is not recommended. However, some experts recommend screening — by stool antigen tests, urea breath testing, or endoscopy — in high-risk asymptomatic people, such as those from countries with a high gastric cancer prevalence and those who have first-degree relatives with gastric cancer. Clinicians should make sure that all H. pylori–positive patients receive adequate eradication therapy.

Trastuzumab Deruxtecan as Second-Line Treatment in HER2-Positive Gastric Cancer[90]

Survival was superior for trastuzumab deruxtecan over paclitaxel plus ramucirumab, confirming it as the preferred treatment. DESTINY-Gastric04 is a globally practice-changing trial. Trastuzumab deruxtecan should be the preferred second-line treatment after gastric cancer progression on trastuzumab-based first-line treatment in patients retaining HER2-positive status.

Trastuzumab deruxtecan is approved in the U.S. for second- or later-line treatment and globally for third- or later-line treatment of human epidermal growth factor receptor 2 (HER2)–positive esophagogastric adenocarcinoma after disease progression on first-line trastuzumab-based treatment. Investigators now report results of an open-label, phase 3 DESTINY-Gastric04 trial of second-line treatment of unresectable or metastatic HER2-positive esophagogastric adenocarcinoma after disease progression on trastuzumab.

Patients with central confirmation of retained HER2-positive status received standard weekly paclitaxel and ramucirumab or trastuzumab deruxtecan every 3 weeks at 6.4

mg/kg. Of the 494 patients treated, 61% had gastric and 39% had gastroesophageal junction primaries, 84% were immunohistochemical (IHC) 3+ and 15% IHC 2+ and in situ hybridization (ISH)–positive, and 25% had experienced disease progression after less than 6 months of first-line therapy.

The primary endpoint of overall survival was superior for trastuzumab deruxtecan compared with paclitaxel–ramucirumab (14.7 vs. 11.4 months; hazard ratio, 0.7), as were progression-free survival (6.7 vs. 5.6 months; HR, 0.74) and objective response (44.3% vs 29.1%). Rates of drug-related serious adverse events for the two treatments were similar, with interstitial lung disease (mostly grade 2; grade 3 in one patient) occurring in 14% of patients treated with trastuzumab deruxtecan.

Should We Add Durvalumab to Perioperative FLOT for Gastric and Gastroesophageal Cancer?[92]

Yes: Durvalumab significantly improved event-free survival when added to perioperative chemotherapy. Adding durvalumab to perioperative FLOT chemotherapy in resectable gastroesophageal adenocarcinoma is the new global standard of care.

For patients with resectable gastric cancer, perioperative chemotherapy with fluorouracil, leucovorin, oxaliplatin, and docetaxel (FLOT) is the standard of care. Given that immune checkpoint inhibitors improve metastatic gastric cancer outcomes after chemotherapy, researchers are studying these agents as add-ons to perioperative chemotherapy in the curative setting. Investigators now report results from a double-blind, placebo-controlled, randomized, multinational phase 3 MATTERHORN trial. Participants received neoadjuvant durvalumab (or placebo) plus perioperative FLOT, surgery, and additional, adjuvant durvalumab (or placebo) to complete 1 year of therapy. Approximately 950 patients with gastric (68%) or gastroesophageal junction (33%) primary adenocarcinomas underwent surgery and were included in the study. Of these, 66% had a primary tumor stage of T3 and 25% T4, and 90% tested positive for PD-L1 expression.

The results showed

- Durvalumab-FLOT (D-FLOT) significantly increased event-free survival (the primary endpoint) (67%) compared with FLOT alone (59%) at 24 months.

- The secondary endpoint of overall survival at 24 months also was significantly better with D-FLOT, 76%, over FLOT, 70%.
- Pathologic complete response was also more common with D-FLOT (19%) compared with FLOT (7%).

The two treatment groups had similar rates of R0 resection, completion of therapy before and after surgery, and grade 3 or 4 treatment-related adverse events (72 with both treatments).

While mature overall survival results are pending, this trial demonstrated durvalumab's superiority in event-free survival and improved pathologic complete response. The differences are clinically meaningful.

Individualizing Endoscopic Surveillance for Barrett's Esophagus[103]

A randomized trial showed no difference in cancer rates or mortality between surveillance and symptom-based endoscopy.

Evidence to support regular surveillance endoscopy for patients with Barrett's esophagus comes mainly from observational studies and expert opinion. Evidence from randomized, controlled trials has been lacking. In a U.K. study, researchers randomized 3500 patients (mean age, 63; 99% with no dysplasia) to surveillance endoscopy every 2 years or to as-needed endoscopy based on symptoms (for example, dysphagia, iron deficiency anemia, weight loss). Patients were followed for a median of 13 years.

About 60% of patients in the as-needed group underwent at least 1 endoscopy, versus 90% of patients in the surveillance group; mean screening intervals were 23 months in the surveillance group and 32 months in the symptom-based group.

Mortality was similar in the two groups (≈20%), as were cancer-related mortality and diagnosis of esophageal adenocarcinoma.

The American Gastroenterological Association incorporated this study in its 2025 Barrett's esophagus screening guideline, which recommends that patients without dysplasia undergo surveillance endoscopy every 3 to 5 years. This study contributed to a growing body of work that supports more individualized approaches for screening patients with Barrett's esophagus

12. PANCREATIC CANCER

Tumor Treating Fields for Locally Advanced Pancreatic Cancer[60]

Overall survival and pain-free survival were both extended when tumor treating fields(TTF) therapy was added to chemotherapy.

Tumor treating fields (TTF) is a noninvasive therapy that uses alternating low-intensity electric fields to inhibit cancer cell proliferation. Investigators reported treatment outcomes in patients with locally advanced unresectable pancreatic adenocarcinoma who received gemcitabine and nab-paclitaxel with or without TTF in an industry-sponsored, open-label phase 3 global trial. Of the 571 participants, most had tumors of the pancreatic head (51%) or body (28%). Nearly half (43%) received treatment in North America, 58% were ECOG PS 1, and only 4% were ECOG 2.

Overall survival (OS) was significantly lengthened with the addition of TTF to chemotherapy over chemotherapy alone (median, 16.2 months vs. 14.2 months; hazard ratio, 0.82), with no significant difference in progression-free survival (PFS; range, 9.3–10.6 months). Although local PFS did not differ appreciably between groups, distant PFS was significantly extended when TTF was added to chemotherapy (13.9 months vs. 11.5 months; HR, 0.74). Pain-free survival was also significantly improved with TTF (15.2 months vs. 9.1 months; HR, 0.74). The most common device-related adverse events — dermatitis, rash, and pruritus — occurred in up to 28% of patients.

13. MELANOMA

Final 10-Year Outcomes with Nivolumab plus Ipilimumab in Advanced Melanoma[69]

The final trial results showed a continued, ongoing survival benefit with nivolumab plus ipilimumab compared to ipilimumab monotherapy, in patients with advanced melanoma.

Previous results from this trial showed longer overall survival after treatment with nivolumab plus ipilimumab or with nivolumab monotherapy than with ipilimumab monotherapy in patients with advanced melanoma. Given that patients with advanced melanoma were living longer than 7.5 years, longer-term data were needed to address new clinically relevant questions.

The investigators randomly assigned patients with previously untreated advanced melanoma, in a 1:1:1 ratio, to one of the following regimens: nivolumab (1 mg per kilogram of body weight) plus ipilimumab (3 mg per kilogram) every 3 weeks for four doses, followed by nivolumab (3 mg per kilogram) every 2 weeks; nivolumab (3 mg per kilogram) every 2 weeks plus placebo; or ipilimumab (3 mg per kilogram) every 3 weeks for four doses plus placebo. Treatment was continued until the occurrence of disease progression, unacceptable toxic effects, or withdrawal of consent. Randomization was stratified according to BRAF mutation status, metastasis stage, and programmed death ligand 1 expression. They reported the final 10-year results of this trial, including results for overall survival and melanoma-specific survival, as well as durability of response.

With a minimum follow-up of 10 years, median overall survival was 71.9 months with nivolumab plus ipilimumab, 36.9 months with nivolumab, and 19.9 months with ipilimumab. The hazard ratio for death was 0.53 (95% confidence interval [CI], 0.44 to 0.65) for nivolumab plus ipilimumab as compared with ipilimumab and was 0.63 (95% CI, 0.52 to 0.76) for nivolumab as compared with ipilimumab. Median melanoma-specific survival was more than 120 months with nivolumab plus ipilimumab (not reached, with 37% of the patients alive at the end of the trial), 49.4 months with nivolumab, and 21.9 months with ipilimumab. Among patients who had been alive and progression-free at 3 years, 10-year melanoma-specific survival was 96% with nivolumab plus ipilimumab, 97% with nivolumab, and 88% with ipilimumab.

Nivolumab for Resected Stage III or IV Melanoma at 9 Years[146]

The 9-year final data support a sustained finding of longer recurrence-free survival with nivolumab than with ipilimumab.

In the CheckMate 238 trial, patients with resected stage IIIB–C or stage IV melanoma who were treated with nivolumab had longer recurrence-free survival than those who received ipilimumab. Data were needed on longer-term survival.

The investigators randomly assigned patients in a 1:1 ratio to receive an intravenous infusion of nivolumab (at a dose of 3 mg per kilogram of body weight every 2 weeks) or ipilimumab (at a dose of 10 mg per kilogram every 3 weeks for four doses, then every 12 weeks) for up to 1 year or until disease recurrence or the occurrence of unacceptable toxic effects. Randomization was stratified according to disease stage and status with respect to programmed cell death ligand 1. The primary end point was recurrence-free survival; secondary end points included overall and distant metastasis-free survival and safety.

At a minimum follow-up of nearly 9 years (107 months), the median duration of recurrence-free survival was 61.1 months with nivolumab and 24.2 months with ipilimumab (hazard ratio for recurrence or death, 0.76; 95% confidence interval [CI], 0.63 to 0.90); 9-year recurrence-free survival was 44% and 37%, respectively. The median duration of distant metastasis–free survival in patients with stage III melanoma was more than 9 years with nivolumab and 83.8 months with ipilimumab, with 9-year survival of 54% and 48%, respectively (hazard ratio for distant metastasis or death, 0.81; 95% CI, 0.65 to 1.00). The median overall survival was more than 9 years in both trial groups, with 9-year survival of 69% in the nivolumab group and 65% in the ipilimumab group (hazard ratio for death, 0.88; 95.03% CI, 0.69 to 1.11). The rates of death from melanoma at 9 years were 26% with nivolumab and 30% with ipilimumab (hazard ratio, 0.87; 95% CI, 0.67 to 1.13). Subsequent systemic therapy was administered to fewer patients in the nivolumab group than in the ipilimumab group (37.3% vs. 44.6%). No new late adverse events were reported.

14. NON-MELANOMA SKIN CANCERS

Adjuvant Cemiplimab for Cutaneous Squamous-Cell Carcinoma: Making the Case[75]

In a phase 3, placebo-controlled trial involving patients with high-risk cutaneous squamous cell carcinoma (cSCC), cemiplimab yielded longer disease-free survival.

Cutaneous squamous-cell carcinoma (cSCC) is a localized disease that can be cured surgically in most patients. However, about 5% develop nodal or distant metastases in association with more aggressive disease. These invesigators present data from C-POST, the first randomized trial of adjuvant immunotherapy with cemiplimab (which targets programmed death 1 [PD-1]) in patients with resected high-risk cSCC.

A total of 415 participants were assigned to receive either cemiplimab or placebo for up to 48 weeks with a median follow-up of 24 months. Patients were generally well matched for high-risk characteristics between groups. Regarding the primary endpoint of disease-free survival (DFS), the hazard ratio for recurrence or death was 0.32 - an indication of benefit for recipients of immunotherapy. Estimated DFS at 24 months' follow-up was 87% (cemiplimab) versus 64% (placebo). Toxicities were as expected for this class of drugs, with grade 3 adverse event rates reported as 24% (cemiplimab) and 14% (placebo).

This study makes a compelling case for adjuvant cemiplimab in the treatment of patients with resectable high-risk cSCC. While potentially practice-changing, the findings are unsurprising given the high response rates (~50%) seen with anti–PD-1 agents in metastatic or unresectable cSCC. Moreover, a nonrandomized, phase 2 study demonstrated impressive activity for neoadjuvant cemiplimab with a pathologic complete response rate of 51%, further demonstrating immunotherapy's potent activity in this disease setting. Given the precedent seen in melanoma for the superiority of neoadjuvant anti–PD-1 therapy, it is likely that neoadjuvant therapy will be afforded priority in the right patient population, with adjuvant therapy serving as a solid alternative approach — and with either option clearly superior to surgery alone.

Resolution of Squamous-Cell Carcinoma by Restoring T-Cell Receptor Signaling by Allogeneic HSC Transplantation[129]

Restoration of the integrity of TCR signaling by allogeneic hematopoietic-cell transplantation led to the resolution of all HPV-related diseases in this patient.

Cutaneous squamous-cell carcinoma (SCC) is primarily caused by oncogenesis mediated by ultraviolet radiation, and β-human papillomavirus (β-HPV) is believed to be a facilitator that is dispensable for the maintenance of cutaneous SCC. In this study the investigators described a woman with benign and malignant HPV-related diseases that included a recurrent, unresectable, invasive cutaneous SCC with β-HPV19 genomic integration in the context of germline pathogenic mutations in ZAP70, an adapter required for T-cell receptor (TCR) signal transduction. Restoration of the integrity of TCR signaling by allogeneic hematopoietic-cell transplantation led to the resolution of all HPV-related diseases, thereby revealing a direct role of β-HPV in skin carcinogenesis in hosts with defective adaptive T-cell responses.

Although the causative and prognostic roles of ultraviolet exposure, Fitzpatrick skin type, age, and sex in cutaneous SCC have been well defined and even incorporated into risk-prediction models, the contribution of immunosurveillance against cutaneous β-human papillomaviruses (β-HPVs) in the pathogenesis of cutaneous SCC remains unclear. Whereas a direct oncogenic role has been firmly established for mucosal α-HPVs that are integrated into the host genome in mucosal SCC (i.e., in the anogenital, oropharyngeal, or respiratory tract) and constitutively express the E6/E7 viral oncogenes, cutaneous β-HPVs are believed to have an indirect role as facilitators of skin carcinogenesis. β-HPVs appear to be relevant at an early stage of carcinogenesis by enabling the accumulation of ultraviolet-induced DNA mutations. However, these β-HPVs have not been found to be stably transcribed in samples of established cutaneous SCC and, therefore, are considered to be dispensable in the maintenance of a frankly malignant phenotype. In addition, although the role of immunosurveillance in skin carcinogenesis is inferred by the high prevalence of cutaneous SCC in immunocompromised hosts and by the clinical response to checkpoint inhibitors in patients with a high mutational burden, the contribution of immunologic escape to viral or ultraviolet-mediated neoantigens in skin carcinogenesis remains uncertain.

Inborn errors of immunity can help to decipher the role of HPVs and specific immunologic functions in skin and mucosal carcinogenesis. In this study the investigators reorted on the immunopathogenesis and management of recurrent, treatment-refractory, invasive cutaneous SCC associated with a β-HPV in the context of defective proximal T-cell receptor (TCR) signaling owing to germline variants in the gene encoding the zeta chain of the TCR-associated protein kinase 70 (ZAP70). The regression of multiple benign and recurrent malignant HPV-related lesions after restoration of HPV-specific T-cell responses following hematopoietic-cell transplantation (HCT) illustrates the role of adaptive T-cell functions and the implications of integrated ablative and immunotherapeutic approaches for severe HPV-related diseases.

The patient provided written informed consent for enrollment in three clinical studies and was seen at the National Institutes of Health (NIH) Clinical Center for all study visits at screening, baseline, follow-up, and ad hoc evaluations for incidental clinical needs. The experimental methods included flow cytometric analysis for T-cell immunophenotyping, functional analysis of T-cell activation and proliferation, analysis of HPV-specific T-cell responses, and assessment of DNA repair, as well as Western blot analysis of ZAP70 signaling and histologic and molecular analysis of the cutaneous SCC for HPV genotyping, single-base substitution analysis, and identification of somatic variants in cancer-relevant genes.

15. ENDOMETRIAL CANCER

Hormone Therapy or Hysterectomy for Endometrial Cancer: Balancing Fertility Preservation Against Survival[61]

In women younger than 40 with early-stage endometrial cancer, survival was comparable after progestin therapy or hysterectomy; in those aged 40 to 49, risk for death was higher after progestin therapy.

Fertility-preserving hormonal therapy is an increasingly accepted option among young women with early-stage endometrial cancer — but the long-term effects on survival are unclear? The researchers conducted a retrospective observational study of almost 16,000 women (age range, 18–49 years) with stage I, grade 1 or 2 endometrial cancer (stage I is limited to the uterus; grade 1 or 2 is associated with less-aggressive endometrioid histology). Approximately 1,200 women received uterus-preserving progestin therapy and 14,700 underwent hysterectomy.

Throughout 5 years' follow-up among patients younger than 40, survival did not differ between those who received progestins (98.2%) or hysterectomy (98.5%). However, among those aged 40 to 49, survival was 90.4% with progestin treatment and 99.4% with hysterectomy — thus, the risk for death was significantly higher in association with progestin treatment (hazard ratio, 4.9).

For patients younger than 40 with early-stage endometrial cancer who want to become pregnant during the next year, progestin treatment and assessment of the response to therapy with endometrial sampling is advised. If progestin therapy is successful, the patient should pursue an attempt at pregnancy immediately. For women aged 40 and older with early-stage endometrial cancer, hysterectomy is strongly recommend. If fertility-preserving progestin therapy is planned for these patients, it should be limited to the period of time needed to achieve a pregnancy; After thar, hysterectomy should be performed.

16. CERVICAL CANCER

Cervical Cancer Mortality in Women Younger Than 25[30]

In this age group, cervical cancer mortality has decreased dramatically in recent years.

Cervical cancer incidence among young women in the U.S. has declined during the past decade, largely attributable to the successful introduction of the human papillomavirus (HPV) vaccine in 2006. Using national health statistics, researchers analyzed trends in cervical cancer mortality among women younger than 25 between 1992 and 2021.

The number of cervical cancer deaths in this age group decreased from 55 (in 1992–1994) to 13 (in 2019–2021); in total, 398 deaths occurred. The rate of decline accelerated across this 30-year interval, particularly after 2015.

This study's design did not allow for causal inference (because data on HPV vaccination status were not available), but previous research has shown that HPV vaccination lowers cervical cancer incidence. The authors noted that one quarter of U.S. adolescents have not received even one dose of the HPV vaccine.

Coming Soon: At-Home Cervical Cancer Screening?[84]

We are one step closer to an easily accessible in-home screening option. The shift toward primary human papillomavirus (HPV)–based screening for cervical cancer screening has also shifted our focus toward more comfortable alternatives to speculum-based exams. In 2024, the U.S. FDA approved an in-office, self-collected vaginal swab — and recently has authorized the first at-home option. In two recent studies, researchers compared results of self-collected and clinician-collected specimens and examined uptake of self-collection.

In a multisite U.S. study, 582 women self-collected HPV swabs in their physicians' offices, prior to speculum-based clinician sampling. Self-collected samples had >95% agreement with clinician-collected samples for detecting high-risk HPV — thus meeting screening standards.

In a study of 2,500 people (94% from under-screened, under-represented minorities) in Texas, participants were randomized to receive one of the following: A telephone reminder about clinic-based screening only, a reminder plus a mailed self-collection kit, or a reminder with a kit plus a follow-up call. At 6 months, receipt of a self-collection kit — whether alone or with follow up — increased the likelihood of completing screening compared with a reminder alone (41% and 48% vs. 17%).

An at-home testing option has strong potential to reach those who are unable or unwilling to use current office-based screening options. These test kits (Teal Wand and others) currently can be prescribed and shipped only via the telehealth route (starting in California). Clinicians currently are not able to order them directly.

Sentinel-Lymph-Node Biopsy Alone or with Lymphadenectomy in Cervical Cancer[127]

In patients with early-stage cervical cancer, sentinel-lymph-node biopsy alone was noninferior to lymphadenectomy with respect to disease-free survival and was associated with fewer complications.

In this multicenter, randomized, noninferiority trial, the investigators enrolled patients with cervical cancer that was stage IA1 (with lymphovascular invasion), IA2, IB1, or IIA1 according to 2009 International Federation of Gynecology and Obstetrics criteria. Sentinel-lymph-node biopsy was performed at the time of surgery and was followed by examination of frozen sections. Patients who had negative sentinel lymph nodes were intraoperatively assigned in a 1:1 ratio not to undergo pelvic lymphadenectomy (the biopsy-only group) or to undergo lymphadenectomy (the lymphadenectomy group). All patients underwent hysterectomy, and adjuvant therapy was provided according to a unified protocol. The primary end point was disease-free survival at 3 years, with a prespecified noninferiority margin of 5 percentage points in the upper limit of the confidence interval for the difference between the lymphadenectomy group and the biopsy-only group. Secondary end points included retroperitoneal nodal recurrence, cancer-specific survival, and surgical complications.

A total of 838 patients underwent randomization: 420 patients were assigned to the biopsy-only group and 418 to the lymphadenectomy group. The median follow-up was 62.8 months. The 3-year disease-free survival was 94.6% in the lymphadenectomy group and 96.9% in the biopsy-only group (difference, −2.3 percentage points; 95% confidence interval [CI], −5.0 to 0.5; P<0.001 for noninferiority); the 3-year cancer-specific survival was 99.2% in the biopsy-only group and 97.8% in the lymphadenectomy group (hazard ratio for death from cancer in competing-risks analysis, 0.37; 95% CI, 0.15 to 0.95). Retroperitoneal nodal recurrences occurred in no patients in the biopsy-only group and in 9 patients (2.2%) in the lymphadenectomy group. The biopsy-only group had a lower incidence of lymphocyst than the lymphadenectomy group (8.3% vs. 22.0%; P<0.001), as well as a lower incidence of lymphedema (5.2% vs. 19.1%; P<0.001), paresthesia (4.0% vs. 8.4%; P=0.009), and pain (2.6% vs. 7.9%; P=0.001).

17. THYROID CANCER

Do GLP-1–Receptor Agonists Increase Risk for Thyroid Cancer?[148]

A large, international cohort study of patients with type 2 diabetes found no significant short-term association between GLP-1–receptor agonist use and thyroid cancer risk, but long-term effects require further investigation.

Glucagon-like peptide-1–receptor agonists (GLP-1–RAs) are widely used for type 2 diabetes and obesity management, but concerns have emerged regarding their potential association with thyroid cancer, given the increased GLP-1 receptor expression in thyroid cancer cells and preclinical findings of C-cell malignancies in rodents. While some observational studies suggest an increased risk, others report no association.

To investigate this potential association in patients with type 2 diabetes, researchers analyzed population-based databases from six countries and identified roughly 100,000 GLP-1–RA users and 2.5 million dipeptidyl peptidase-4 inhibitor (DPP-4i) users. The median follow-up period ranged from 1.8 to 3.0 years for GLP-1–RA users and from 2.8 to 6.8 years for DPP-4i users.

In mortality-adjusted Cox regression models, the pooled weighted hazard ratio for thyroid cancer among GLP-1–RA users compared with DPP-4i users was 0.81 (95% CI, 0.59–1.12), indicating no significant increase in thyroid cancer risk associated with GLP-1–RA use. Additionally, analyses considering cumulative GLP-1–RA doses did not reveal an elevated risk. Subgroup analyses for thyroid cancer subtypes (e.g., medullary thyroid cancer) were not feasible due to a low number of these outcomes.

These findings from the largest population study on this question so far suggest that GLP-1–RA use does not increase the risk for thyroid cancer in the short term, which is consistent with results from other recently reported observational studies using DPP-4i or sodium–glucose cotransporter-2 inhibitor as active comparators (Diabetes Obes Metab 2024; 26:108; BMJ 2024; 385:e078225). While this may offer reassurance to patients and clinicians regarding the safety of GLP-1–RAs, the relatively short follow-up periods in these studies limit conclusions about long-term risks.

18. BILIARY TRACT CANCER

Does Adding Nab-Paclitaxel to First-Line Chemotherapy in Biliary Cancer Improve Survival?[36]

The answer is no. Furthermore, it increases treatment-related toxicity.

The combination of gemcitabine and cisplatin (GC) is standard chemotherapy for advanced biliary cancer and is usually used together with durvalumab or pembrolizumab for first-line therapy. In 2019, a phase II study demonstrated positive results with the addition of nanoparticle albumen-bound (nab)-paclitaxel to first-line GC in advanced biliary cancer. This study has completed a randomized, open-label, phase 3 trial of this regimen, with overall survival (OS) as the primary endpoint. Patients received standard GC either alone or in combination with nab-paclitaxel

(100 mg/m^2 on days 1 and 8 of a 21-day cycle). Of 441 patients, 55% were female, 67% had intrahepatic cholangiocarcinoma, and 73% had metastatic disease.

Patients receiving nab-paclitaxel had a higher overall response rate than those receiving GC alone (31% vs. 21%), but no significant differences were seen in OS (median, 14 vs. 13.6 months; hazard ratio, 0.91) or progression-free survival (7.5 vs. 6.3 months; HR, 0.89). The addition of nab-paclitaxel was associated with higher rates of treatment-related grade 3/4 adverse events, both hematologic (60% vs. 45%) and nonhematologic. Treatment-related grade 5 events were much more common with the addition of nab-paclitaxel (7 patients) than with GC alone (1 patient).

These results indicate that adding a taxane to GC does not improve survival in advanced biliary cancer and that it increases treatment-related toxicity. GC plus either durvalumab or pembrolizumab remains the standard of care.

19. HEPATOCELLULAR CARCINOMA

Adding Lenvatinib plus Pembrolizumab to Transarterial Chemoembolization for Hepatocellular Carcinoma[40]

The combination improved progression-free survival and objective response rate but not overall survival.

Immunotherapy combinations, including tremelimumab plus durvalumab, ipilimumab plus nivolumab, and atezolizumab plus bevacizumab, have demonstrated superiority over tyrosine kinase inhibitors (TKIs) in the treatment of advanced hepatocellular cancer (HCC) and are considered first-line therapy in that setting. In liver-confined HCC, the addition of single-agent TKIs to regional therapy has led to mixed and largely negative results compared with regional therapy alone.

Investigators reported results from the LEAP-012 trial, an industry-sponsored, global, phase 3 study in which patients with unresectable nonmetastatic HCC were randomized to receive transarterial chemoembolization (TACE) in combination with either lenvatinib plus pembrolizumab (LP) or dual placebo. TACE (whether conventional or with drug-eluting beads) was limited to two treatments per tumor. Of the 480 study participants, 72% were Asian, and the cause of HCC was hepatitis B in 62%, alcohol in 46%, and hepatitis C in 17%.

Progression-free survival was significantly better with LP than with placebo (median, 14.6 vs. 10.0 months; hazard ratio; 0.66; P=0.0002), as was objective response rate (47% vs. 33%; P=0.0005). However, no significant difference was seen in overall survival (HR; 0.80, P=0.087), which, at 24 months, was 75% for the LP group and 69% for the placebo group. Grade 3/4 treatment-related serious adverse events occurred in 71% of the LP group compared with 32% of the placebo group.

Although the addition of LP to TACE improved progression-free survival and objective response rate in this trial, it did not improve overall survival. These results mirror those of LEAP-002, in which LP failed to improve survival in advanced HCC compared with lenvatinib alone.

Does Radiation Therapy Improve Survival in Hepatocellular Carcinoma Compared with Sorafenib Alone?[39]

The answer is yes, but whether it will be a beneficial add-on to newer, more effective systemic regimens remains to be seen.

Sorafenib was once standard first-line treatment for inoperable or metastatic hepatocellular cancer (HCC) but has since been replaced by combination immunotherapy or by immunotherapy combined with bevacizumab. Prior to that shift, these investigators initiated an open-label, randomized, phase 3 trial to evaluate whether adding stereotactic body radiotherapy (SBRT) to first-line sorafenib improved overall survival (OS) in patients with Child-Pugh A liver function and HCC not amenable to resection, ablation, or transarterial chemoembolization.

Patients assigned to sorafenib alone received 400 mg twice daily. Those assigned to SBRT and sorafenib received SBRT dosed at 27.5 to 50 Gy in 5 fractions over 5 to 15 days, followed by sorafenib 200 mg twice daily starting 1 to 5 days after radiotherapy and then escalated to 400 mg twice daily as tolerated. Of 177 patients, 49% had clinical stage T3b disease, 74% had macrovascular invasion, 41% had hepatitis C, and 19% had hepatitis B with or without hepatitis C; the median sum of HCC diameter was 7.8 cm. Median follow-up was 13.2 months.

Median OS was 15.8 months with the addition of SBRT and 12.3 months with sorafenib alone, a difference that reached statistical significance only after multivariate adjustment (hazard ratio, 0.72; 95% CI, 0.52–0.99). Progression-free survival was improved with SBRT (median, 9.2 vs. 5.5 months; HR, 0.55; 95% CI, 0.40–0.75), as was response rate (38% vs. 9%). Grade 3/4 treatment-related adverse events occurred in 34% of patients receiving SBRT and 6% of those receiving sorafenib alone.

This trial indicates that adding SBRT to systemic therapy in HCC may improve response, progression-free survival, and OS compared with sorafenib alone. Future trials need to assess the potential benefit of adding SBRT to newer, more effective systemic regimens for liver-confined HCC.

Nivolumab plus ipilimumab showed a significant overall survival benefit versus lenvatinib or sorafenib and manageable safety in patients with previously untreated unresectable hepatocellular carcinoma[87]

Immune checkpoint inhibitor–based regimens are standard first-line treatment for unresectable hepatocellular cancer (HCC). Such regimens include bevacizumab plus atezolizumab, tremelimumab plus durvalumab, and now, based on new trial results, nivolumab plus ipilimumab.

CheckMate 9DW was an open-label, phase 3 trial in which 668 patients with unresectable HCC were randomized to receive either nivolumab (1 mg/kg) plus ipilimumab (3 mg/kg) every 3 weeks for four treatments, followed by monthly nivolumab (480 mg; IPI/NIVO), or the investigator's choice of either lenvatinib or sorafenib (LS). Patients were predominantly male (82%), with about 40% treated in Asia and another 40% in Europe or North America; 34% had hepatitis B and 28% had hepatitis C.

The results were:

- During a median 3 years' follow-up, the IPI/NIVO group had a median overall survival of 23.7 months compared with 20.6 months in the LS group, a significant difference. The IPI/NIVO group had higher rates of overall survival at both 24 months (49% vs. 39%) and 36 months (38% vs. 24%).

- Early treatment-related deaths occurred in 12 patients receiving IPI/NIVO and 3 receiving LS.
- Median progression-free survival (PFS) was similar in the two groups (approximately 9 months), but the PFS rate at 24 months was higher with IPI/NIVO than with LS (28% vs. 12%).
- Patients receiving IPI/NIVO had a significantly higher response rate than those receiving LS (36% vs. 13%) and a longer median duration of response (30.4 vs. 12.9 months).
- Both groups had about a 40% rate of grade 3/4 treatment-related adverse events.

IPI/NIVO is now a standard-of-care treatment for unresectable HCC in the first-line setting. Given the high rate of treatment-related deaths in this study, some clinicians may opt to use the potentially better-tolerated schedule of nivolumab (3 mg/kg) combined with ipilimumab (1 mg/kg).

The Advent of Perioperative Immunotherapy in Early-Stage Hepatocellular Carcinoma[108]

Perioperative camrelizumab plus rivoceranib more than doubles event-free survival compared with surgery alone in select patients with hepatocellular carcinoma.

Even with optimal surgical resection, up to 80% of patients with early-stage hepatocellular carcinoma (HCC) experience recurrence, particularly those with bulky tumors or vascular invasion. Numerous adjuvant therapies, including atezolizumab and bevacizumab, have failed to improve outcomes. The role for perioperative immunotherapy remains under-investigated. A multicenter, randomized, phase 2/3 (CARES-009) trial, conducted in China, compared perioperative camrelizumab (a PD-1 inhibitor) plus rivoceranib (an antiangiogenic tyrosine kinase inhibitor) with surgery alone. Camrelizumab and rivoceranib are not FDA-approved. The study included 294 patients with early-stage HCC. The primary end point was event-free survival (EFS). Approximately 75% of patients had hepatitis B liver disease with more metabolic dysfunction–associated steatohepatitis and hepatitis C liver disease.

- Perioperative camrelizumab plus rivoceranib significantly improved EFS compared with surgery alone (median: 42 vs. 19 months).

- Nearly all patients underwent definitive surgical resection (92% vs. 98%), and all were R0 (negative margin) resections.
- Grade ≥3 treatment-related adverse events were significantly more common with perioperative therapy (38% vs. 0%), including 2 deaths during neoadjuvant therapy.

The opportunity to improve event-free survival in early-stage hepatocellular carcinoma by almost 2 years is of interest. The EFS results were striking, but the mature overall survival data will be critical to determine if the efficacy of this regimen justifies its toxicity.

20. NEUROENDOCRINE TUMORS

Phase 3 Trial of Cabozantinib to Treat Advanced Neuroendocrine Tumors[43]

The investigators enrolled two independent cohorts of patients — those with extrapancreatic neuroendocrine tumors and those with pancreatic neuroendocrine tumors — who had received peptide receptor radionuclide therapy or targeted therapy or both. Patients were randomly assigned in a 2:1 ratio to receive cabozantinib at a dose of 60 mg daily or placebo. The primary end point was progression-free survival as assessed by blinded independent central review. Key secondary end points included objective response, overall survival, and safety.

In the cohort of 203 patients with extrapancreatic neuroendocrine tumors, the median progression-free survival with cabozantinib was 8.4 months, as compared with 3.9 months with placebo (stratified hazard ratio for progression or death, 0.38; 95% confidence interval [CI], 0.25 to 0.59; P<0.001). In the cohort of 95 patients with pancreatic neuroendocrine tumors, the median progression-free survival with cabozantinib was 13.8 months, as compared with 4.4 months with placebo (stratified hazard ratio, 0.23; 95% CI, 0.12 to 0.42; P<0.001). The incidence of confirmed objective response with cabozantinib was 5% and 19% among patients with extrapancreatic and pancreatic neuroendocrine tumors, respectively, as compared with 0% with placebo. Grade 3 or higher adverse events were noted in 62 to 65% of the patients treated with cabozantinib, as compared with 23 to 27% of the patients who received placebo. Common treatment-related adverse events of grade 3 or higher included hypertension, fatigue, diarrhea, and thromboembolic events.

The authors concluded that cabozantinib, as compared with placebo, significantly improved progression-free survival in patients with previously treated, progressive advanced extrapancreatic or pancreatic neuroendocrine tumors. Adverse events were consistent with the known side-effect profile of cabozantinib.

Belzutifan for Advanced Pheochromocytoma or Paraganglioma[111]

Belzutifan showed antitumor activity with durable responses in participants with advanced pheochromocytoma or paraganglioma.

Pheochromocytoma and paraganglioma are neoplasms originating in the adrenal medulla and extra-adrenal paraganglia, respectively. Most cases of metastatic pheochromocytoma and paraganglioma are driven by dysregulation of the hypoxia-inducible factor 2α (HIF-2α) pathway. Belzutifan is a HIF-2α inhibitor that may provide antitumor activity in patients with advanced pheochromocytoma or paraganglioma.

The researchers conducted a phase 2, international, single-group trial involving 72 participants with locally advanced or metastatic pheochromocytoma or paraganglioma that was not amenable to surgery or curative-intent treatment. Participants received belzutifan at a dose of 120 mg once daily until the occurrence of progression, unacceptable toxic effects, or withdrawal from the trial. The primary end point was confirmed objective response (complete or partial response) as assessed by blinded independent central review. Secondary and other key end points included the duration of response, disease control, progression-free survival as assessed by blinded independent central review, overall survival, safety, and a reduction from baseline in antihypertensive medication.

At a median follow-up of 30.2 months (range, 23.3 to 37.6), the percentage of participants with a confirmed objective response was 26% (95% confidence interval [CI], 17 to 38) and the percentage of participants with disease control was 85% (95% CI, 74 to 92). The median duration of response was 20.4 months (95% CI, 8.3 to not reached), with a median duration of progression-free survival of 22.3 months (95% CI, 13.8 to not reached). Overall survival was 76% at 24 months. Among the 60 participants who were receiving antihypertensive medications, 19 (32%) had a reduction of at least 50% in the total daily dose of at least one antihypertensive medication for at least 6 months after starting treatment with belzutifan. Treatment-related adverse events occurred in 71 participants (99%); anemia of grade 3 was noted in 22% of the participants. Eight participants (11%) had treatment-related serious adverse events.

21. CARCINOMA OF UNKNOWN PRIMARY SITE[135]

Cancer of unknown primary site is an ever-evolving disease entity and one of the most challenging diagnoses to manage in oncology. The term "cancer of unknown primary site" encompasses a diverse group of histologically confirmed cancers that have metastasized by the time of presentation, with the primary site of origin eluding detection despite a standard diagnostic workup. Patients with cancer of unknown primary site use more health care resources, including more investigations, emergency visits, and hospitalizations, than patients with known primary sites.

Although immunophenotyping is the mainstay of diagnosis, recent advances have led to the integration of molecular profiling in predicting the tissue of origin and identifying targetable alterations in the management of cancer of unknown primary site. Both site-specific therapy (treatment of a putative primary site) and empirical chemotherapy (with a platinum-based cytotoxic regimen) are acceptable options for treatment.

The overall prognosis for patients with cancer of unknown primary site remains poor. Cancer of unknown primary site accounts for 2 to 4% of all cancers. The American Cancer Society estimates that approximately 37,370 new cases of cancer of unknown primary site will be diagnosed in the United States in 2025. Worldwide, incidence rates have been declining and range between 2 and 15 cases per 100,000 person-years. Factors that have possibly contributed to this decreasing trend include enhanced diagnostic methods together with the expanded use of molecular profiling that can more accurately identify the primary site, improved quality of reporting, and better identification of key differential diagnostic elements, such as recurrence of antecedent cancers.

Key Subsets within Cancer of Unknown Primary Site and the Therapeutic Implications.

Although the pathophysiologic mechanisms underlying cancer of unknown primary site remain unclear, a broad postulate has emerged, fostered by our understanding of the biologic underpinnings of metastases from known primary sites.

Development of Cancer of Unknown Primary Site.

The diagnosis of cancer of unknown primary site relies on a comprehensive workup aimed at evaluating for the presence of any primary lesion. However, the extent of diagnostic testing may be restricted by resource constraints, coexisting medical conditions, and the therapeutic window (the urgency of treatment dictated by the extent and pace of disease and the symptom burden). The clinical evaluation begins with obtaining a careful history, including a review of family and personal history of previous cancers. A physical examination and baseline laboratory evaluation can help direct further workup. All patients should undergo imaging (ideally a CT scan with the use of contrast material) of the chest, abdomen, and pelvis. The use of adjunct diagnostic methods, such as PET scan, magnetic resonance imaging, mammography, testicular ultrasonography (in young men with midline lymphadenopathy), or invasive procedures (upper endoscopy, colonoscopy, bronchoscopy, laryngoscopy, or cystoscopy), should be guided by symptoms, imaging, or pathological findings indicative of a primary origin.

Diagnostic Workup for Patients with Cancer of Unknown Primary Site:

Carcinoma: cytokeratin (AE1/3, EMA, Pankeratin)

Lymphoma: CD45

Squamous cell carcinoma: CK5/6, p40, p63

Germ cell tumors: Oct3/4, PLAP, SALL4

Lung cancer: CK7, napsin A, TTF1

Sarcoma: desmin, vermentin

Gastroesophageal cancer: CK7, CK20

Bile duct cancer: CEA, CK7, CK19, CK20

Colo-rectal cancer: CDX2, CK20, SATB2

Pancreas cancer: CA19,9, CDX2, CK7

Kidney cancer: PAX2, PAX8, WT1

Mesothelioma: CK5/6, D2-40, WT1

Prostate cancer: NKX3.1, P5045, PAP, PSA

Endometrial cancer: CK7, ER, PAX8, PR

Ovarian cancer: CK7, ER, PAX8, WT!

Melanoma: HMB-45, melan A, MITF-1, S100, SOX10

Urothelial cancer: CK7, CK 20, GATA3, thrombomodulin, uroplakin

Neuroendocrine carcinoma or neuroendocrine features: CD56, chromogranin A, synaptophysin

Immunophenotyping

Light microscopic examination of tumor tissue with immunophenotyping remains the mainstay in the diagnosis of cancer of unknown primary site. The accuracy of immunohistochemical testing for diagnosing tissue type is high, especially if adequate tumor tissue is assessed. When possible, a core-needle biopsy is preferred to preserve features of tissue architecture that assist with diagnosis. Pathologists use an average of 8.8 immunostains (range, 0 to 20) in evaluating metastatic tumors, and nearly two thirds of patients with cancer of unknown primary site will have insufficient tissue left for molecular profiling during the course of their clinical care. Despite this heavy reliance on immunohistochemical testing, its accuracy in identifying a primary organ is limited, especially in cases of poorly differentiated tumors. Because no one immunostain is pathognomonic of the tissue of origin, a panel of tests performed in a stepwise fashion may be warranted. The use of deep-learning methods for determining the tissue of origin may be the next frontier in the pathology of cancer of unknown primary site.

Molecular Profiling for the Prediction of Tissue of Origin

Molecular profiling in cancer of unknown primary site has been used to predict a putative primary site (tissue-of-origin profiling) and to identify targetable genomic alterations (genomic profiling) amenable to targeted therapies. Several tissue-of-origin assays have been developed on the premise that cancer of unknown primary site and metastases from known primary sites are alike. Therefore, a biomarker set can be generated on the basis of commonalities in genomic, transcriptomic, and epigenetic profiles with the use of a discovery cohort of known primary sites to predict the probability of a match between the signature of cancer of unknown primary site and that of cancer of known primary site. Various strategies that use RNA, microRNA, DNA, and methylation coupled with machine learning have been developed, with accuracy in predicting the tissue of origin ranging from 65 to 99%.39 Among these strategies, only gene-expression profiling has been evaluated in randomized trials, with mixed results.

Principles of Treatment

The goal of treatment in most patients with cancer of unknown primary site is largely palliative owing to the disseminated nature of the disease, except for a small subpopulation of patients who present with single-site or limited metastatic disease. In these patients, a multidisciplinary approach incorporating radiation therapy or surgery can be potentially curative.

Treatment Algorithm for Management of Cancer of Unknown Primary Site

Patients with cancer of unknown primary site who present with a characteristic, recognizable, clinicopathological pattern that is analogous to specific known primary cancers can be treated according to guidelines pertaining to those specific tumors, a treatment approach that simply emulates a site-specific approach to therapy for cancer of unknown primary site. However, most patients with cancer of unknown primary site do not have a typical presentation. In these cases, clinicopathological clues can be used to discern a putative primary site, despite the clear absence of a primary lesion. Tissue-of-origin profiling for discerning primary sites may also be helpful. For cancer of unknown primary site with a discernible primary site, preference should be given to first-line site-specific therapy, which mirrors the standard care for the corresponding metastatic cancer of known primary site.

Several retrospective studies and prospective trials have investigated the benefit of site-specific therapy over empirical chemotherapy with conflicting results. Two multicenter trials, the Next Generation Sequencing for Patients with Cancer of

Unknown Primary Site (CUP-NGS) trial (involving 130 patients) and the Groupe d'Etude Français des Carcinomes de site Primitif Inconnu-04 (GEFCAPI-04) trial (involving 243 patients), randomly assigned patients with newly diagnosed cancer of unknown primary site to site-specific therapy (on the basis of gene-expression profiling to predict the primary site) or to empirical chemotherapy (carboplatin plus paclitaxel in the CUP-NGS trial and gemcitabine plus cisplatin in the GEFCAPI-04 trial). Neither trial showed superiority of site-specific therapy over empirical chemotherapy. Overall survival at 1 year was 44.0% in the site-specific therapy group and 54.9% in the empirical therapy group (P=0.26) in the CUP-NGS trial and was 41.3% and 40.7%, respectively (P=0.71), in the GEFCAPI-04 trial. The corresponding median progression-free survival was 5.1 months and 4.8 months (P=0.55) in the CUP-NGS trial and 4.6 months and 5.3 months (P=0.71) in the GEFCAPI-04 trial.

Summary of Studies Evaluating the Role of Site-Specific Therapy as Compared with Empirical Therapy in Cancer of Unknown Primary Site

Contrary to these trials, the single-center, randomized Fudan CUP-001 trial (involving 182 patients) showed superiority of site-specific therapy guided by gene-expression profiling over platinum-based empirical chemotherapy (plus a taxane or gemcitabine). The median progression-free survival was 9.6 months with site-specific therapy and 6.6 months with empirical chemotherapy (P=0.017). Heterogeneity of the population and improved systemic therapies, specifically the incorporation of targeted therapies and immunotherapy (in nearly 45% of patients) in the experimental group, may have affected this advantage with respect to progression-free survival.

Empirical Chemotherapy

A meta-analysis of five studies (three observational studies and two randomized trials. The most common empirical chemotherapy used in practice was a combination of a platinum agent (carboplatin or cisplatin) with either paclitaxel or gemcitabine. Other regimens comprising gemcitabine plus docetaxel and a fluorouracil-based therapy are also used. A meta-analysis of 32 studies (including 7 randomized trials) evaluating 42 regimens did not show clear superiority of any one regimen.

Molecularly Guided Targeted Therapy

Biomarker-driven therapies, specifically those with proven efficacy regardless of the specific tissue or organ where the cancer originated are endorsed by guidelines for cancer of unknown primary site. Genomic aberrations are common in cancer of unknown primary site, and response to targeted therapies has been documented in case series and nonrandomized studies. The CUPISCO trial (involving 436 patients) evaluated the clinical benefit of incorporating molecular profiling to identify targetable genomic alterations; the trial used tumor tissue, a blood-based assay, or both. In this trial, patients with cancer of unknown primary site who had disease control after three cycles of standard first-line platinum-based chemotherapy and were randomly assigned to receive therapy guided by molecular profiling had progression-free survival that was 6 weeks longer than those who were assigned to continued chemotherapy (median, 6.1 vs. 4.4 months; P=0.008), even though less than one third of the patients assigned to molecular profiling–guided therapy had an actionable target.

Areas of Uncertainty

The rarity of cancer of unknown primary site and the paucity of research amplify the uncertainty in the treatment of patients with this morbid orphan disease. Although the debate on effective therapy for cancer of unknown primary site is shifting toward site-specific and molecularly guided therapies, high-level evidence regarding improvement in outcomes with these therapies over treatment guided by standard clinicopathological assessment is lacking.

Guidelines

The National Comprehensive Cancer Network (NCCN), the National Institute for Health and Care Excellence (NICE), and the European Society for Medical Oncology (ESMO) publish and regularly update guidelines focused on the evaluation and treatment of patients with cancer of unknown primary site.

22. NON-HODGKIN LYMPHOMA

Refractory B cell lymphomas: towards a New Frontier in CAR T-Cell Therapy[6]

An innovative pluripotent stem cell–derived CAR natural killer cell showed both safety and efficacy in refractory B-cell lymphomas.

Chimeric antigen receptor (CAR) T-cell therapy is an effective option for relapsed B-cell lymphoma, but access to treatment may be limited due to rapid disease progression, the time required for CAR T-cell manufacture, and geographic barriers for patients needing management at specialized centers. Investigators now report a novel CD19-targeted natural killer (NK) cell CAR (FT596) derived from an allogeneic induced pluripotent stem cell that was engineered to include an immunoglobulin Fc receptor (CD16), to enhance tumor cell targeting when co-administered with rituximab, and an interleukin-15 ligand/receptor fusion protein, to mitigate the need for exogenous cytokine support.

This multicenter, phase 1 trial tested multiple FT596 cell dose levels administered with or without rituximab to 86 patients with relapsed or refractory B-cell lymphomas, including 33 who had received prior autologous CAR T-cell therapy. Thirty-nine patients received a second dose of FT596. Toxicities included grade 1–2 cytopenias, with only one dose-limiting toxicity (thrombocytopenia). Ten patients had grade 1–2 cytokine release syndrome, and none had neurotoxicity or graft-versus-host disease. There were no FT596-related adverse events that caused treatment discontinuation or death.

All 13 patients with follicular lymphoma responded, including 85% complete remissions (CR); a third of the 32 patients with large B-cell lymphoma responded, 25% achieved CR. Responses also were achieved in other B-cell lymphoma subtypes and in 30% of patients who had received prior CAR T-cell therapy. With a median follow-up of 26 months, no patient in CR had experienced disease progression.

FT596 is a novel allogeneic cellular therapeutic that can be delivered as a cryopreserved, off-the-shelf product in the outpatient setting. These early results show a favorable toxicity profile and encouraging activity, as well as the promise of overcoming some limitations of current CAR T-cell therapy for B-cell lymphoma and, potentially, for other blood cancers and solid tumors.

CAR T-Cell Therapy for Large B-Cell Lymphoma: Promise and Precautions[26]

One third of patients with relapsed/refractory disease remained in remission at 5 years, but late non-relapse mortality due to infection and second malignancies were common.

Anti-CD19 CAR T-cell therapy is potentially curative for patients with relapsed or refractory large B-cell lymphoma (R/R LBCL), although long-term outcomes are not yet fully known. In this study, investigators reported updated, 5-year results of a multicenter retrospective analysis of axicabtagene ciloleucel (axi-cel) therapy in 275 patients who had received at least two prior lines of therapy. Bridging therapy was allowed prior to CAR T-cell administration; 43% of patients would not have been eligible for the registrational clinical trial that led to FDA approval of axi-cel.

Findings at a median follow-up of 58 months were as follows:

1. The overall response rate was 82%, with complete response in 64%; three early deaths were related to CAR T-cell–associated toxicities.
2. The 5-year progression-free survival was 29%, and 5-year overall survival was 40%.
3. Of 118 progressions or relapses, 102 occurred within 2 years of CAR T-cell infusion, with only 5 after year 3.
4. Nonrelapse mortality was 16.2% at 5 years, mostly due to infections and second primary malignancies, and continued to occur throughout the years following the CAR T-cell product infusion.
5. Patients aged 60 and older had a lower incidence of lymphoma relapse, but higher non-relapse mortality, than younger patients.

This analysis confirmed CAR T-cell therapy as a curative approach in R/R LBCL, while identifying prolonged immunodeficiency and severe infections as well as late second primary cancers. About half of the latter were treatment-related myeloid malignancies, at least in part due to prior chemotherapy. The shift of CAR T-cell therapy to patients with first relapse and less-extensive prior lymphoma therapy, and better approaches to immune reconstitution, may mitigate some late non-relapse mortality events.

Strengthening Induction Therapy for Aggressive B-Cell Lymphoma[50]

Adding glofitamab to R-CHOP or Pola-R-CHP yielded a response rate of 100% in younger patients with high-risk large B-cell lymphoma

Glofitamab is a bispecific T-cell engaging monoclonal antibody with single-agent activity in relapsed or refractory large B-cell lymphoma (LBCL). Now, investigators have assessed the safety and efficacy of combining glofitamab with R-CHOP (rituximab, cyclophosphamide, doxorubicin, vincristine, and prednisone) or Pola-R-CHP (polatuzumab, rituximab, cyclophosphamide, doxorubicin, and prednisone) in patients with high-risk international prognostic index scores, double-hit (DH) LBCL, or both. (DHL is an uncommon subtype of diffuse large B-cell lymphoma (DLBCL), making up about 5% of DLBCL cases. In DHL, the lymphoma cells have mutations or rearrangements of two significant genes – the MYC gene and either the BCL2 or BCL6 genes. Most lymphoma cells have a rearrangement on one only or none of these genes). (Glofitamab was initiated with stepped-up dosing in cycle 2; after completing induction chemotherapy, an additional two cycles of single-agent glofitamab were given. The primary endpoint was safety; response and survival outcomes were secondary endpoints.

Of 80 eligible patients, 11% had DH LBCL and 74% received an initial cycle of R-CHOP; 96% completed all planned treatment cycles. In each arm, approximately 40% of patients had peripheral neuropathy and approximately 20% had cytokine release syndrome. The overall best response rate was 100%; one patient in each arm had progressive disease. At a median follow-up of 17 months postinduction, the estimated 24-month progression-free survival was 86% and overall survival was 92% in both arms. Overall, 8 patients experienced disease progression, with 2 deaths occurring while in remission.

These promising results confirm that glofitamab can be safely added to R-CHOP or Pola-R-CHP, and support further pursuit of prospective trials that incorporate glofitamab or other bispecific antibodies into front-line therapy for high-risk aggressive B-cell lymphomas.

Epstein-Barr Virus as a Cause of Cancer in Recipients of Kidney Transplantation[27]

More than one in five EBV-negative kidney transplant recipients developed post-transplant lymphoproliferative disease within 3 years of receiving organs from EBV-seropositive donors.

In a retrospective cohort study, investigators matched 104 high-risk (EBV Donor+/Recipient−) adults to 312 low-risk (EBV Recipient+) adults who had received kidney transplants. Most recipients underwent induction immunosuppression with thymoglobulin. During the 3-year post-transplant follow-up period, post-transplant lymphoproliferative disease (PTLD) developed in 22% of high-risk patients at a median of 202 days after transplant. No cases were identified among EBV R+ or D−/R− individuals. EBV D+/R− status was significantly associated with graft failure (hazard ratio, 2.21); risk for death was also higher (HR, 2.19), but not statistically significantly so.

PTLD is a significant cause of death in solid organ transplant recipients, and the one-in-five chances of developing this cancer in high-risk patients emphasizes the need for preventive strategies and rigorous diagnostic efforts whenever symptoms suggest PTLD. Accordingly, these investigators now monitor EBV DNA in blood samples, as an indicator of viral load, frequently in high-risk patients and modulate immunosuppression as appropriate, even though data are scant to guide this approach.

CAR+ T-Cell Lymphoma after Cilta-cel Therapy for Relapsed or Refractory Myeloma[42]

Chimeric antigen receptor (CAR) T-cell therapies have shown remarkable efficacy against hematologic malignant disease, but secondary T-cell malignant neoplasms represent a newly identified classwide danger signal. As of December 2023, the Food and Drug Administration (FDA) was aware of 22 cases in which T-cell malignant neoplasms developed after the administration of approved CAR T-cell therapies with more than 27,000 doses of such therapies given in the United States. CAR transgenes have been detected in malignant clones in three patients for whom data were available; however, clinical and genomic details have not been published, and the number of patients who had samples available for testing was not stated.

Ciltacabtagene autoleucel (cilta-cel) is an FDA-approved anti–B-cell maturation antigen–directed CAR T-cell therapy that is produced by means of lentiviral transduction. In the phase 3, randomized CARTITUDE-4 trial involving patients with lenalidomide-refractory multiple myeloma who had received one to three previous lines of therapy, cilta-cel significantly improved progression-free survival as compared with standard care.

In this paper the authors presented the clinicogenomic characterization of two patients from this trial in whom peripheral T-cell lymphoma (PTCL)–not otherwise specified (PTCL-NOS, a malignant monoclonal T-cell lymphoproliferation with CAR transgene integration and expression) developed after they had received cilta-cel therapy. In the absence of direct evidence, the role of insertional mutagenesis to the development of T-cell lymphoma is currently unclear.

The authors referred to this condition as CAR transgenic T-cell lymphoproliferative neoplasm (CTTLN).

CD4+ T-Cell Lymphoma Harboring a Chimeric Antigen Receptor Integration in TP53[43]

The authors reported a case of a T-cell lymphoma harboring a lentiviral integration in a known tumor suppressor, TP53, which developed in a patient with multiple myeloma after B-cell maturation antigen (BCMA) CAR T-cell therapy.

The exact causes of secondary T-cell cancers are uncertain, but one potential mechanism is insertional mutagenesis in T cells. In most T-cell cancers after CAR T-cell therapy reported to date, the vector integrations occurred in genes of unclear oncogenic potential, which made it difficult to establish a causal association with tumorigenesis. The authors described a case of T-cell lymphoma of the gastrointestinal (GI) tract occurring several weeks after treatment with ciltacabtagene autoleucel (cilta-cel), a BCMA CAR T-cell therapy for multiple myeloma. This tumor appeared to be a cancer associated with integration of the CAR vector within a canonical tumor-suppressor gene (TP53, which encodes tumor protein p53).

A 72-year-old woman with relapsed, triple-class–refractory IgA kappa multiple myeloma and a high-risk cytogenetic profile had received four lines of myeloma-directed therapy (including two autologous hematopoietic stem-cell transplants) before treatment with fludarabine–cyclophosphamide lymphodepleting chemotherapy followed by cilta-cel, an autologous BCMA-specific 4-1BB/CD3-zeta CAR T-cell therapy. The treatment course was notable for grade 1 cytokine release syndrome and resulted in a minimal residual disease (MRD)–negative complete remission by 1 month after cilta-cel therapy.

Approximately 2 months after infusion, the patient reported new and persistent nausea, vomiting, anorexia, and intractable watery, nonbloody diarrhea and was ultimately hospitalized. Evaluation for an infectious cause was negative, and computed tomography of the abdomen and pelvis did not show any clinically significant abnormalities. She underwent upper endoscopic and flexible sigmoidoscopic evaluations that revealed a normal-appearing esophagus, stomach, proximal duodenum, and colon, with biopsy samples obtained during both procedures.

The histopathological findings of the upper endoscopy were believed to be compatible with a potential immune-mediated enterocolitis of unclear cause. The patient received various treatments, including glucocorticoids, tacrolimus, and high-dose infliximab but did not have a sustained response. The treatment course was complicated by cytomegalovirus reactivation resulting in treatment with ganciclovir. Eventually, ruxolitinib was started at a dose of 5 mg orally twice daily, then increased to 10 mg orally twice daily. Over the course of 2 weeks, her appetite improved and the diarrhea decreased in frequency, leading to planning for potential hospital discharge. However, shortly before discharge, clinical signs of sepsis developed with blood cultures growing *Stenotrophomonas maltophilia* and *Streptococcus mitis*, Despite broad-spectrum antibiotic therapy, her condition worsened with septic shock and acute respiratory failure. In concert with her family, the clinical team pursued comfort care measures, and the patient died with her family at her side.

The authors used an in-house digital droplet polymerase-chain-reaction assay for the detection of the cilta-cel CAR constructs in blood and other biologic specimens. CAR was detected in high abundance in DNA extracted from the patient's duodenal-biopsy samples.

These findings prompted a pathological re-examination of the original duodenal-biopsy samples Immunohistochemical analysis showed a dense lymphocytic infiltration of the lamina propria positive for T-cell receptor (TCR) α, CD3, CD4, and granzyme B but which did not express TRBC1 chain (a marker for expression of a T-cell antigen receptor constant beta chain) or CD8. No lamina propria plasma cells were detected by BCMA staining. The pathological diagnosis was reclassified as an indolent CD4+ T-cell lymphoma or lymphoproliferative disorder of the GI tract.

T cell repertoire sequencing of the duodenal-biopsy samples revealed a dominant TCR Vβ11-02 clone representing 83.59% of productive TCR sequences, a finding consistent with a clonal CAR+ lymphoproliferative process. CAR integration-site analysis of the duodenal-biopsy samples identified two dominant insertion sites: the first integrated in reverse orientation in the first intron (chromosome 17: 7683124) of TP53 and the second in positive orientation in the first intron (chromosome 22: 20025368) of the gene encoding transport and golgi organization 2 homolog (TANGO2). The two insertions were found at similar frequencies (29% and 23%, respectively); these findings, in conjunction with a single dominant clone on TCR sequencing, were most consistent with a single clone bearing CAR in both TP53 and TANGO2.

The p53 protein expression in the duodenal-biopsy samples was assessed with the use of immunohistochemical analysis and showed physiologic expression in the crypt epithelial cells. However, the majority (90%) of T cells showed dim or absent p53, a finding consistent with reduced expression in clonal T cells.

Whole-exome sequencing of the duodenal-biopsy samples identified 23 additional mutations relative to a pre-infusion blood sample. A missense mutation in the gene encoding suppressor of cytokine signaling 1 (SOCS1), with a serine-to-phenylalanine substitution (pS206F) in the "SOCS box" domain that regulates protein degradation was found. SOCS1 is a negative regulator of Janus kinase (JAK)–signal transducer and activator of transcription (STAT) signalling, and previous studies have established phosphorylated STAT 3 (pSTAT3) as a readout for active JAK–STAT signalling. Immunohistochemical analysis for pSTAT3 showed strong staining in 80 to 90% of T cells, a finding consistent with reduced SOCS1 activity leading to increased JAK–STAT signalling.

To understand the kinetics of clonal emergence, the authors performed TCR sequencing on serial peripheral-blood samples obtained before and after CAR infusion. The TCR Vβ11-02 clone was detected at a frequency of 16.99% of TCR sequences at day 74 after infusion, coincident with the onset of clinical symptoms. The same clone was detectable at a frequency of 0.01% of sequences on day 28 but was not detectable at any previous time point either before or after infusion (days 3 and 14 after CAR T-cell infusion). In addition, a high-frequency TCR Vβ27-01 clone was detected in the peripheral blood (29.34%) on day 74 after infusion but not at any previous time points. This clone was detected at low abundance (<2%) in the duodenal-biopsy samples.

To better characterize clonal progression in the blood, the authors performed whole-genome sequencing on blood samples obtained before infusion (on day −58) and after infusion (on days 14 and 74). We detected a Y284* nonsense mutation in the gene encoding DNA methyltransferase 3 alpha (DNMT3A) at a variable allele frequency (VAF) of 7.6% in the pre-infusion sample, which represented pretreatment clonal hematopoiesis in this patient. The DNMT3A alteration was stably present at approximately 10% VAF at both day 14 and 74 but was below the limit of detection in the post-infusion GI lymphoma sample. No additional mutations or structural variants in TP53 were detected. A total of 22 of 23 variants, including the SOCS1 pS206F mutation, were identified by at least two reads in the day 74 whole-genome sequencing of peripheral blood, coincident with the emergence of the Vβ11-02 clone The SBS1 and SBS5 "clock-like" mutational signatures were predominant in both the duodenal-biopsy samples and the day 74 peripheral-blood samples.

To further characterize the consequence of genetic alterations, the authors performed single-cell RNA sequencing with single-cell VDJ (variable, diversity, and joining) sequencing on approximately 18,000 cells from peripheral-blood samples pooled from three time points (days 14, 28, and 74). The TCR Vβ11-02 clone clustered independently and represented approximately 3% of all cells.

This is not the first report of a CAR T-cell–derived lymphoproliferative process occurring in the gut after treatment with cilta-cel. However, this study described a lymphoma harboring a CAR transgene integration into a common cancer-associated gene.

The authors identified integration of a lentiviral vector in an antisense orientation in the first intron of TP53. Lentiviral vectors show preference for insertion in transcription units, which may disrupt regulatory sequences necessary for gene expression or generate alternate isoforms through splice donor or acceptor sites in the retroviral vector sequence. The results of immunohistochemical analysis and single-cell RNA sequencing were consistent with decreased TP53 transcription and reduced p53 expression in clonal T cells bearing the TP53-integrated CAR vector.

Whether a monoallelic TP53 CAR vector integration confers a predisposition to transformation is unclear. An additional integration in TP53 was detected as a single event in the duodenal-biopsy samples obtained from the patient but was not associated with clonal expansion. Furthermore, in a study involving 58 patients treated with CD19 CAR T cells, 19 unique integration sites were found in the TP53 transcription unit, and none were associated with clonal expansion, which suggests that monoallelic TP53 integration alone is not sufficient to transform CAR T cells. Therefore, a search was made to identify alternative factors that may have contributed to oncogenesis.

A second dominant insertion was detected in TANGO2, a gene with poorly described function that is associated with developmental disorders but has no known role in oncogenesis. Its transcriptional expression was maintained in our clone.

The authors also detected a mutation in SOCS1, a known tumor suppressor that regulates cytokine signalling through JAK–STAT pathways. The substitution occurred in the degradation-regulating "SOCS box" domain at a site that has previously been implicated in large B-cell lymphoma. Immunohistochemical analysis confirmed JAK–STAT pathway activation, and the patient had a notable clinical improvement after initiating treatment with ruxolitinib, a JAK2 inhibitor.
Both TP53 and SOCS1 alterations are commonly identified and can co-occur in patients with peripheral T-cell lymphoma.

This case showed that preexisting clonal mutations may not necessarily contribute to, and are not required for, all scenarios of CAR T-cell malignancies.

Enhanced CAR T-Cell Therapy for Lymphoma after Previous Failure[134]

In this small study, huCART19-IL18 had a safety profile consistent with other CAR T-cell treatments and showed promising efficacy at low cell doses in patients with lymphoma after the failure of previous anti-CD19 CAR T-cell therapy.

Chimeric antigen receptor (CAR) T cells targeting CD19 have transformed the treatment of B-cell cancers, but many patients do not have a long-term remission. The investigators designed an anti-CD19 enhanced (armored) CAR T-cell product (huCART19-IL18) that secretes interleukin-18 to enhance antitumor activity.

In this study, they assessed the safety, feasibility, and preliminary efficacy of huCART19-IL18 in patients with relapsed or refractory lymphoma after previous anti-CD19 CAR T-cell therapy. Using a 3-day manufacturing process, we administered huCART19-IL18–positive cells in doses ranging from 3×10^6 to 3×10^8.

A total of 21 patients received huCART19-IL18. Cytokine release syndrome occurred in 62% of the patients (47% with grade 1 or 2), and immune effector-cell–associated neurotoxicity syndrome occurred in 14% (all grade 1 or 2). No unexpected adverse events were observed. Robust CAR T-cell expansion was detected across all dose levels. At 3 months after infusion, a complete or partial response was seen in 81% of the patients (90% confidence interval [CI], 62 to 93) and a complete response in 52% (90% CI, 33 to 71). With a median follow-up of 17.5 months (range, 3 to 34), the median duration of response was 9.6 months (90% CI, 5.5 to not reached).

An Improved Therapeutic for Cutaneous T-Cell Lymphoma[141]

One third of patients with relapsed or refractory disease responded to the reformulated therapeutic fusion protein denileukin diftitox-cxdl. (Denileukin diftitox-cxdl, a recombinant DNA-derived fusion protein, is an IL2-receptor-directed cytotoxin).

Limited treatment options are available for advanced-stage cutaneous T-cell lymphoma (CTCL). From 1999 to 2014, the fusion protein denileukin diftitox (DD) was available in the U.S. for CTCL treatment but then was withdrawn and reformulated to improve purity and bioactivity. Investigators have now reported on the reformulation, DD-cxdl, which, like its predecessor, links diphtheria toxin fragments to interleukin 2 (IL-2) and then binds to tumor cells expressing the IL-2 receptor, with subsequent intracellular toxin release and tumor-cell death.

In this multicenter, phase 3, single-arm trial, 69 patients with relapsed or refractory stage IA–IIIB mycosis fungoides or Sézary syndrome and at least one prior systemic therapy received DD-cxdl (9 μg/kg/d intravenously on 5 consecutive days in 21-day cycles for 8 cycles). Those with a response (measured in skin, blood, lymph nodes, and viscera) could continue longer.

Patients had a median age of 64 years (range, 28–87) and a median of four prior systemic therapies (range, 1–18). The overall response rate (primary endpoint) was 36.2%, with complete responses in 8.7%; treatment responses occurred within 2 months, and median response duration was 8.9 months. More than 80% of patients had cutaneous responses, with about half showing at least a 50% decrease in skin lesions. Infusion reactions occurred in 74% of patients (almost all grade 1/2 and in the first 2 cycles), hepatotoxicity in 36% (grade 3/4 in 4–9%), and capillary leak syndrome in 20% (most in the first 3 cycles; grade 3/4 in 6%). Five patients discontinued treatment due to toxicity.

Based on these results, the FDA has approved DD-cxdl for patients with relapsed CTCL and prior systemic therapy; a "black box" warning for capillary leak syndrome was included. DD-cxdl is an important agent with a novel mechanism of action and should be considered for patients with relapsed CTCL.

23. HODGKIN LYMPHOMA

A New Standard Treatment for Older Individuals with Hodgkin Lymphoma[76]

For patients aged ≥60 with advanced-stage disease, front-line nivolumab plus AVD chemotherapy yielded better outcomes than brentuximab vedotin plus AVD.

Patients over 60 with classic Hodgkin lymphoma (cHL) have worse treatment responses and outcomes than younger patients due to comorbidities, poor tolerance of therapy, and differences in HL biology. In the S1826 study, investigators assessed 6 cycles of the immune checkpoint inhibitor nivolumab (N) plus AVD (doxorubicin, vinblastine, and dacarbazine) versus brentuximab vedotin (BV) plus AVD in previously untreated patients with advanced-stage cHL and stratified by age group.

Findings for participants aged ≥60 years:

- Two-year progression-free survival was significantly better for N-AVD (89%) than BV-AVD (64%); 2-year overall survival was 96% vs. 85%.

- Adverse events (including peripheral neuropathy) were more common with BV-AVD, and dose reductions were not necessary in 26% (BV-AVD) vs. 69% (N-AVD) of participants.
- Progression or relapse occurred in 8% (N-AVD) vs. 18% (BV-AVD) of patients; non-relapse mortality was 6% vs. 16%.

Biologic Classification of Hodgkin Lymphoma: A New Era for an Old Disease?[8]

Next-generation sequencing of circulating tumor DNA revealed clinically relevant subtypes and a tool to monitor minimal residual disease.

For over 50 years the management of Hodgkin lymphoma (HL) has been based on stage at presentation and more recently by initial treatment response on interim PET scanning. Unlike with other lymphomas, histomorphology has not guided therapy, except for nodular lymphocyte-predominant HL. These investigators reported a retrospective analysis of circulating plasma tumor DNA sequencing, gene expression profiling, and tumor microenvironment (TME) profiling in blood and tissue samples from patients enrolled in trials for previously untreated advanced-stage HL (German Hodgkin Study Group HL21) and early-stage unfavorable HL (NIVAHL). Samples and patient outcomes from a frontline pediatric HL trial (EuroNet-PHL-C2) served as the validation cohort. Minimal residual disease (MRD) was assessed after two cycles of combination chemotherapy for patients in the HL21 trial.

- Three biologic HL subtypes were identified and confirmed in the external validation cohort:
- Inflammatory immune escape HL — frequent chromosomal copy number variations, including 9p24.1 amplification containing PD-L1
- Virally-driven HL — enrichment of HL-associated Epstein-Barr virus and/or human herpesvirus 6
- Oncogene-driven HL — mutations in NFkB and interferon signalling, MHC-1-Ag presentation, and cell cycle regulation.
- TME characterization also showed three distinct gene expression profiles that correlated with the biologic subtypes, as did TME immune cell composition.
- Three-year progression-free survival was improved after two treatment cycles in MRD-negative versus MRD-positive patients with inflammatory immune escape HL (91.5% vs. 55.5%) and virally driven HL (95.1% vs. 72.5%),

whereas outcomes were similar between MRD-negative and MRD-positive patients with oncogene-driven HL (3-year PFS >90%). The identification of distinct biologic subtypes in HL opens a new frontier into understanding mechanisms of lymphomagenesis, individual patient risk stratification and clinical characteristics, and treatment outcomes. If these findings are confirmed in additional retrospective as well as prospective analyses, a new era for risk-adapted treatment and prognosis will occur. Further analysis is of special interest for patients receiving front-line brentuximab vedotin-based regimens and immune checkpoint inhibitor-based regimens.

24. CHRONIC LYMPHOCYTIC LEUKEMIA

Observe or Treat Early-Stage Chronic Lymphocytic Leukemia?[13]

In patients with Binet stage A disease and risk factors for early progression, ibrutinib was associated with delayed onset of symptoms but no survival benefit.

In the chemotherapy era, clinicians observed patients with asymptomatic, early-stage chronic lymphocytic leukemia (CLL) and did not give anti-CLL therapy until treatment was indicated by symptom onset or clinically significant disease progression. Investigators from Germany have reported long-term outcomes with a Bruton tyrosine kinase (BTK) inhibitor in patients with Binet stage A CLL and intermediate-to-high risk for early progression according to a multifactorial risk score.

In this prospective, multicenter, double-blind, phase 3 trial, 363 patients received oral ibrutinib (420 mg daily) or placebo until disease progression or treatment intolerance. Another 152 patients with low-risk CLL underwent watchful waiting and regular monitoring of disease status. Findings at a median follow-up of 69 months showed that

1. Progression to symptomatic disease was significantly delayed with ibrutinib compared with placebo (21.4% vs. 51.4%; hazard ratio, 0.276)
2. Ibrutinib showed no 5-year overall survival (OS) benefit compared with placebo (93.3% and 93.6%, respectively). Five-year OS in the low-risk, watch-and-wait group was 97.9%.

3. One of 12 deaths in the ibrutinib arm and 4 of 14 deaths in the placebo arm were due to CLL.

Toxicity-related events, including arrhythmias, hypertension, and bleeding events, were numerically more frequent in ibrutinib-treated patients. Testing the traditional approach to asymptomatic CLL in the era of targeted therapeutics endorsed this watch-and-wait strategy, even in higher-risk patients. Thus, watch and wait remains the standard of care, with the caveat that more-frequent symptom monitoring, examinations, and blood counts are warranted in patients at elevated risk for early progression.

An Emerging Option for Treatment of Richter Transformation[20]

The immune checkpoint inhibitor atezolizumab in combination with venetoclax and obinutuzumab provided high responses in CLL/SLL with large B-cell lymphoma transformation.

Diffuse large B-cell lymphoma (DLBCL) arising in patients with preexisting chronic lymphocytic leukemia/small lymphocytic lymphoma (CLL/SLL), known as Richter transformation, is associated with poor response and short survival following immunochemotherapy. In this study investigators reported a prospective, multicenter, phase 2 trial of the programmed cell death-ligand 1 (PD-L1) inhibitor atezolizumab (A), the BCL2 inhibitor venetoclax (V), and the anti-CD20 antibody obinutuzumab (O) in patients with documented CLL/SLL, biopsy-proven DLBCL, no prior treatment with study agents, and no prior DLBC-directed therapy. Patients received AVO in cycles 1 to 8, AV in cycles 9 to 18, and single-agent V in cycles 19 to 35.

The findings were:

- Of the 28 patients enrolled, 19 (67.9%) achieved partial or complete response by the end of AVO cycle 6 (the primary endpoint); four patients progressed before cycle 6 and two did not achieve response at cycle 6 restaging.
- Nineteen patients continued therapy, with six completing cycle 35.
- With a median follow-up of 16.8 months, the 12-month progression-free survival was 42.9% and overall survival 64.3%; 8 of 19 responding patients had ongoing response at 24 months.

- Toxicities included neutropenia and five treatment-related infections (two fatal due to sepsis and fungal pneumonia). Six patients (21%) had immune-related adverse events, but none required treatment discontinuation; no tumor lysis syndrome occurred.

Acalabrutinib Combinations as Initial Therapy for Chronic Lymphocytic Leukemia[35]

Fixed-duration acalabrutinib plus venetoclax, with or without obinutuzumab, outperformed chemoimmunotherapy in patients without TP53 mutation or deletion.

Frontline treatment of chronic lymphocytic leukemia (CLL) with a Bruton tyrosine kinase inhibitor (BTKi) has largely replaced chemoimmunotherapy, with BTKi therapy typically continued until disease progression or unacceptable toxicity occurs. In this study researchers reported a multinational, phase 3 trial comparing fixed-duration acalabrutinib combinations against chemoimmunotherapy in 867 previously untreated patients with CLL. Patients were randomized to 28-day cycles of the BTKi acalabrutinib (A; twice daily, cycles 1–14) plus the B-cell lymphoma-2 inhibitor venetoclax (V; cycles 2–14), or the same regimen plus the anti-CD20 antibody obinutuzumab (O; cycles 2–7), or investigator's choice of 6 cycles of bendamustine-rituximab or fludarabine-cyclophosphamide-rituximab. Patients with TP53 mutation or deletion were excluded, as were those >65 years old with CIRS-Geriatric scores >6.

With a median follow-up of 40.8 months, estimated 36-month progression-free survival (PFS) was significantly improved with AV or AVO versus chemoimmunotherapy (76.5% and 83.1% vs. 66.5%). The 3-year overall survival (OS) was significantly improved with AV versus chemoimmunotherapy (94.1% vs. 85.9%). PFS was improved with AVO versus AV in patients with IGHV-unmutated CLL. Atrial fibrillation of any grade occurred in <1% of the AV and chemoimmunotherapy arms and 2.1% of the AVO arm. Second primary cancers were diagnosed in 5.2% and 4.2% of the AV and AVO arms versus 0.8% of the chemoimmunotherapy arm. Grade 3 or higher infections were more frequent with AVO. Deaths from any cause, including COVID-19 infection, were less common with AV (n=18) than with AVO (n=37) or chemoimmunotherapy (n=42).

In this planned interim analysis of the AMPLIFY trial, AV and AVO significantly improved PFS versus chemoimmunotherapy in fit patients with CLL lacking TP53 aberrations. AVO showed the highest rate of undetectable measurable residual disease as well as improved responses in IGHV-unmutated CLL, albeit with more frequent severe infections and a higher mortality rate than AV. Ongoing follow-up is needed for OS, as is response to second-line therapy following use of doublet- or triplet-targeted agents in the front line.

Measurable Residual Disease–Guided Therapy for Chronic Lymphocytic Leukemia[66]

An interim analysis of progression-free survival in this study showed that ibrutinib–venetoclax was superior to fludarabine–cyclophosphamide–rituximab (FCR) among patients with chronic lymphocytic leukemia (CLL). Whether ibrutinib–venetoclax is more effective than ibrutinib alone is unclear. With extended follow-up and increased enrolment, this trial showed that undetectable MRD and extended progression-free survival were more common with ibrutinib–venetoclax than with ibrutinib alone or FCR. The results for overall survival were also consistent with a benefit of ibrutinib–venetoclax.

In this phase 3, multicenter, open-label trial, the investigators randomly assigned patients with CLL to receive ibrutinib–venetoclax, ibrutinib alone, or FCR. The primary end points were undetectable measurable residual disease (MRD) in bone marrow within 2 years in the ibrutinib–venetoclax group as compared with the ibrutinib-alone group and progression-free survival in the ibrutinib–venetoclax group compared with the FCR group. A powered secondary end point was progression-free survival in the ibrutinib–venetoclax group as compared with the ibrutinib-alone group. Other secondary end points included overall survival.

A total of 172 of the 260 participants (66.2%) in the ibrutinib–venetoclax group had undetectable MRD in bone marrow within 2 years, as compared with none of the 263 participants in the ibrutinib-alone group (P<0.001) and 127 of the 263 participants (48.3%) in the FCR group. With a median follow-up of 62.2 months, disease progression or death occurred in 18 participants (6.9%) in the ibrutinib–venetoclax group, as compared with 59 (22.4%) in the ibrutinib-alone group (hazard ratio, 0.29; 95% confidence interval [CI], 0.17 to 0.49; P<0.001) and 112 (42.6%) in the FCR group (hazard ratio, 0.13; 95% CI, 0.08 to 0.21; P<0.001). Progression-free survival at 5 years was 93.9% with ibrutinib–venetoclax, 79.0% with ibrutinib alone, and 58.1% with FCR. Death occurred in 11 participants (4.2%) in the ibrutinib–venetoclax group, compared with 26 (9.9%) in the ibrutinib-alone group (hazard ratio, 0.41; 95% CI, 0.20 to 0.83) and 39 (14.8%) in the FCR group (hazard ratio, 0.26; 95% CI, 0.13 to 0.50). Sudden death occurred in 3, 8, and 4 participants in the ibrutinib–venetoclax, ibrutinib-alone, and FCR groups, respectively.

25. ACUTE LYMPHOBLASTIC LEUKEMIA

A Remodeled CAR T cell for B-Cell Acute Lymphoblastic Leukemia[153]

Obecabtagene autoleucel provided durable responses in patients with relapsed or refractory disease, with low rates of severe immune-related toxicities.

Anti-CD19 chimeric antigen receptor (CAR) T-cell agents are an established treatment for relapsed or refractory B-cell acute lymphoblastic leukemia (R/R B-ALL). Investigators reported a multinational, phase 1b–2 trial of a novel CAR T-cell therapy containing a modified anti-CD19 binding domain designed to decrease cytokine release syndrome (CRS) and immune effector cell–associated neurotoxicity (ICANS) and to enhance CAR T-cell engraftment and persistence. Adults with R/R B-ALL received a split dose of obecabtagene autoleucel (obe-cel) infusion based on bone marrow tumor cell burden prior to the administration of lymphodepleting chemotherapy.

Of 153 patients, 146 (95%) had successful CAR T-cell manufacture and 127 received obe-cel infusions; 18 patients died or had progressive disease before treatment. Over 90% of patients received pre–CAR T-cell bridging chemotherapy. The findings included:

1. Of 94 patients with morphologically evident residual ALL, 55% achieved complete remission (CR), and another 21% had CR with incomplete hematologic recovery.
2. Among 127 patients who received at least one obe-cel infusion, at a median follow-up of 21.5 months, estimated 6-month and 12-month event-free survival was 65.4% and 49.5%, respectively.

3. Grade 3 or higher CRS occurred in 2.4% of patients; grade 3 or higher ICANS occurred in 7.1%.

Obe-cel provided high response rates in patients with R/R B-ALL, with low rates of severe immune-related toxicities; response rates appear comparable to those with currently available CAR T-cell products. Obe-cel CAR T-cells persisted in peripheral blood for a median of 18 months. Ongoing response was quite durable in patients with <5% pretreatment marrow blasts, while patients with >75% blasts had limited responses of short duration. Further analysis of obi-cel as an earlier line of consolidation, and in patients with measurable residual disease, is planned.

Blinatumomab in Standard-Risk B-Cell Acute Lymphoblastic Leukemia in Children[42]

B-cell acute lymphoblastic leukemia (B-cell ALL) is the most common childhood cancer. Despite a high overall cure rate, relapsed B-cell ALL remains a leading cause of cancer-related death among children. The addition of the bispecific T-cell engager molecule blinatumomab (an anti-CD19 and anti-CD3 single-chain molecule) to therapy for newly diagnosed standard-risk (as defined by the National Cancer Institute) B-cell ALL was investigated in a phase 3 trial involving children with newly diagnosed standard-risk B-cell ALL who had an average or higher risk of relapse. Patients were randomly assigned to receive chemotherapy alone or chemotherapy plus two nonsequential 28-day cycles of blinatumomab. The primary end point was disease-free survival.

The data and safety monitoring committee reviewed the results from the first interim efficacy analysis, which included 1,440 patients who had undergone randomization (722 to chemotherapy alone and 718 to blinatumomab and chemotherapy) and recommended early termination of randomization. At a median follow-up of 2.5 years, the estimated 3-year disease-free survival (±SE) was 96.0±1.2% with blinatumomab and chemotherapy and 87.9±2.1% with chemotherapy alone (difference in restricted mean survival time, 72 days; 95% confidence interval, 36 to 108; P<0.001 by stratified log-rank test). The estimated 3-year disease-free survival among patients with an average relapse risk was 97.5±1.3% with blinatumomab and chemotherapy and 90.2±2.3% with chemotherapy alone; among those with a higher relapse risk, the corresponding values were 94.1±2.5% and 84.8±3.8%. Cytokine release syndrome, seizures, and sepsis of grade 3 or higher were rare during blinatumomab cycles, but the overall incidence of nonfatal sepsis and catheter-related infections was significantly higher among patients with an average relapse risk who had been assigned to receive blinatumomab and chemotherapy than among those assigned to receive chemotherapy alone.

The authors concluded that adding blinatumomab to combination chemotherapy in patients with newly diagnosed childhood standard-risk B-cell ALL of average or higher risk of relapse significantly improved disease-free survival.

Ph-Positive Acute Lymphoblastic Leukemia — 25 Years of Progress[136]

In the past 25 years, from 2000 to 2024, a revolution in the management, treatment, and outcome of what used to be the most lethal hematologic cancer: Philadelphia chromosome–positive acute lymphoblastic leukemia (Ph-positive ALL) has occurred. This progress is an illuminating example of how a better understanding of the biology of a disease, the implementation of targeted treatment directed toward the underlying genetic defect, accurate molecular monitoring of the depth of response to treatment, and most recently, the addition of immunotherapy have provided a cure in most affected patients.

How tyrosine kinase inhibitors (TKIs) Have Changed Frontline Treatment of Ph-Positive ALL

In 2001, Druker et al. reported that patients with relapsed or refractory Ph-positive ALL, as well as those with CML in blast crisis, had a response to the first TKI, imatinib. Similar results were described in 2002 by Ottmann et al. The use of TKIs was extended to the frontline treatment of patients with Ph-positive ALL, and in the past 25 years, these agents have revolutionized the management and outcomes of the disease. The more recent contribution to this success has been the addition of immunotherapy - namely, the bispecific monoclonal antibody blinatumomab - to TKI treatment.

Ph-Positive Acute Lymphoblastic Leukemia

Before the advent of tyrosine kinase inhibitors (TKIs), Ph-positive ALL was the hematologic cancer with the worst outcome. Only the few patients who could undergo allogeneic stem-cell transplantation had a chance of long-term survival.

Initially, TKIs were added to conventional intensive chemotherapy. Since this approach had notable toxic effects, reduced-intensity chemotherapy programs, plus TKIs, were used, an approach resulting in improved responses and outcomes, with fewer toxic effects.

First-, second-, and third-generation TKIs have now been used. These studies have shown the feasibility of this approach, with hematologic complete responses in 94 to 100% of adults, irrespective of age, and with limited toxic effects.

The addition of the bispecific monoclonal antibody blinatumomab (an anti-CD19 and anti-CD3 antibody) in consolidation therapy has further improved molecular response and survival.

A total therapy study (LAL1509) was subsequently conducted, with dasatinib plus glucocorticoids in the induction phase, followed by chemotherapy and transplantation in patients who did not have a complete molecular response. Long-term follow-up showed 5-year overall survival of 56.3% and disease-free survival of 47.2%. Again, patients with early molecular responses had the best outcome, and the presence of additional copy number aberrations - IKZF1 associated with CDKN2A/B, PAX5 deletions (so-called IKZF1plus Ph-positive ALL), or both - was the most important unfavorable prognostic factor.

Studies showed that with the frontline use of targeted treatment directed against the genetic lesion of Ph-positive ALL (BCR:ABL1), patients could be spared the toxic effects of systemic chemotherapy. However, the rates of molecular response at the end of the induction phase remained higher when chemotherapy was added to the TKI during induction.

Additional Role of Blinatumomab

A further step forward was represented by the development of the bispecific monoclonal antibody blinatumomab, which targets CD19 — present on virtually all B-lineage ALLs — and the T-cell antigen CD3. An immunotherapeutic strategy involving blinatumomab aimed to activate the patient's T cells against CD19+ leukemic cells. T

The effectiveness of blinatumomab in combination with dasatinib and glucocorticoids as frontline treatment has been reported in older patients with Ph-positive ALL. The recently published long-term follow-up of the dasatinib–blinatumomab D-ALBA protocol showed that at a median follow-up of 53 months, disease-free survival was 75.8%, overall survival was 80.7%, and event-free survival was 74.6%. No events were recorded for the patients who had an early molecular response. With 93.1% of the patients having a molecular response after dasatinib–blinatumomab treatment, half the patients never received chemotherapy or underwent transplantation, and they continued to receive treatment with only a TKI; all the patients who continued to receive only a TKI except one remain in long-term complete hematologic remission. Allogeneic transplantation was performed during the first remission mainly in patients with persistent MRD, and 83.3% of those patients are in continuous complete hematologic remission.

Recommended and Real-Life Strategies for Frontline Treatment in Adults of All Ages with Ph-Positive ALL.

Long-term follow-up in the D-ALBA study shows that today, using frontline induction with dasatinib, followed by consolidation with blinatumomab, survival of 75 to 80% among adults of all ages with Ph-positive ALL can be expected. The percentage of patients with relapsed disease has decreased dramatically. Extramedullary relapses, particularly in the CNS, have been reporte and have led to intensified intrathecal prophylaxis. Genetic predictors of CNS localization are also being sought.

Another open question is the choice of TKI. Preclinical studies have shown that the second-generation TKI, dasatinib, is more potent than imatinib and that the third-generation TKI, ponatinib, is superior to dasatinib. A significantly higher proportion of patients with no MRD was observed in the ponatinib group in the randomized PhALLCON trial comparing ponatinib with imatinib, plus reduced-intensity chemotherapy, as frontline treatment. Approximately 30% of patients have no molecular evidence of MRD after induction treatment with dasatinib alone plus glucocorticoids and the percentage of patients with MRD negativity increases to approximately 45% with ponatinib and glucocorticoids. Long-term follow-up of the ALL2820 protocol will clarify whether the greater immune activation associated with dasatinib–blinatumomab will be counterbalanced by the lower incidence of ABL1 mutations and fewer relapses with the ponatinib–blinatumomab combination.

Another third-generation TKI, olverembatinib, is effective in patients with CML and the T315I mutation. Alone or in combination with other drugs, olverembatinib has shown activity in relapsed or refractory Ph-positive ALL, including activity in patients with the T315I mutation, and olverembatinib-based regimens have recently been used as frontline therapy in patients with Ph-positive ALL. More studies are needed to clarify the exact role of this new TKI in comparison with the other TKIs and to define its safety profile.

On the basis of a phase 3 trial,79 the FDA has recently granted accelerated approval of asciminib, a first-in-class specific allosteric inhibitor of BCR:ABL1, for the treatment of newly diagnosed CML. In combination with dasatinib, this new TKI, which has a different binding site to BCR::ABL1, may also have a role in the frontline management of Ph-positive ALL.80 However, the data have not shown that asciminib is superior to second-generation TKIs. Chimeric antigen receptor T-cell therapy has so far not been widely applied to Ph-positive ALL.

Twenty-five years of advances in the management of Ph-positive ALL have led to consideration of the possibility of stopping treatment. Treatment-free remission is a goal for many patients with CML. The first data on stopping treatment have been reported in retrospective analyses of patients with Ph-positive ALL who were treated with chemotherapy and a TKI, as well as those treated with a TKI plus reduced-dose chemotherapy or with a TKI alone, which suggest that a fixed duration of treatment may also become a reality for patients with Ph-positive ALL.

The possible overlap between CML in lymphoid blast crisis and Ph-positive ALL has been a long-lasting debate. In the presence of a p210 transcript — the hallmark of CML but also present in a proportion of Ph-positive ALL cases — it is difficult to distinguish between the two conditions. Ph-positive ALL may be more heterogeneous than expected. Subtypes with distinct transcriptomic and genomic profiles, which correlate with multilineage or lymphoid-only BCR:ABL1 involvement, have been identified. In the most recent International Consensus Classification of Myeloid Neoplasms and Acute Leukemias, Ph-positive ALL is subcategorized as lymphoid-only involvement or multilineage involvement. Although this difference is of biologic interest and deserves further investigation, the response to treatment appears to be similar in the two subtypes. Cure can be expected in most adults with

Ph-positive ALL, irrespective of age. A subcutaneous formulation of blinatumomab is under active investigation, with encouraging early results.

26. ACUTE PROMYELOCYTIC LEUKEMIA

Collaborative Initiation of Therapy for Patients with Acute Promyelocytic Leukemia[30]

Collaboration between academic and community practices for timely initiation of treatment markedly improved patient survival in the first month after diagnosis.

Acute promyelocytic leukemia (APL) is a rare, acute, and highly curable malignancy, yet up to 30% of patients die early after diagnosis from disease-related bleeding or complications exacerbated by delays in initiation of all-trans retinoic acid (ATRA)–based induction therapy. In an attempt to decrease early mortality to less than 15%, investigators developed an APL management program that involved rapid initiation of ATRA therapy and the use of a simplified induction treatment algorithm. Consultation from APL experts at academic centers was available to the community site providers around the clock from the time of diagnosis and throughout induction therapy. Six academic and 293 community medical centers across the U.S. participated.

Of 201 eligible patients, 62 were treated at academic, 139 at community sites. The median patient age was 53 years (range, 18–91), 26.4% were considered high-risk based on white blood cell count ≥10,000/dL, and 59% were obese. Only six patients (3%) died in the first month after diagnosis, including five who were aged 70 to 81. Five additional deaths occurred in year 1, one from a treatment complication and four unrelated to APL. Of 11 deaths after year 1, four were due to APL relapse.

The dramatic reduction in early mortality establishes a new paradigm for APL treatment: co-management between academic and community practices, thereby overcoming geographic barriers to access for definitive therapy. Notably, patients treated at the community sites, including high-risk patients, had 1-month and 1-year survival outcomes that were equivalent to or improved over those for patients treated at the academic sites.

A Potential New Standard of Care for High-Risk Acute Promyelocytic Leukemia[50, 51]

De-escalated anthracycline dosing in combination with ATRA plus ATO yielded better outcomes than a more chemo-intensive regimen.

Chemotherapy-free induction therapy with all-trans retinoic acid (ATRA) plus arsenic trioxide (ATO) is the standard of care for standard-risk acute promyelocytic leukemia (APML: white blood cell [WBC] count, $\leq 10\times10^9$/L at diagnosis), conferring higher cure rates and lower risk for early mortality from disease-related coagulopathy. High-risk patients have WBC count $>10\times10^9$/L and greater likelihood of relapse and early mortality despite more-intensive chemotherapy plus ATRA. In a phase 3 industry-supported trial, Platzbecker et al. assessed induction with ATRA–ATO and 2 doses of idarubicin in the first cycle followed by consolidation with 4 cycles of ATRA–ATO, versus induction with ATRA plus 4 doses of idarubicin followed by 3 cycles of consolidation with ATRA plus chemotherapy and 2 years of oral maintenance chemotherapy plus ATRA.

Study enrollment closed early due to slow accrual (related to the COVID-19 pandemic), with 133 participants. At a median follow-up of 37 months, 2-year event-free survival (the primary endpoint) was 88% in the ATRA–ATO arm and 71% in the ATRA–chemotherapy arm. Differentiation syndrome during induction and molecular relapse also were both significantly less likely with ATRA–ATO, although overall survival was similar across all participants due to effective salvage therapies.

At most centers a suspected diagnosis of APML necessitates immediate initiation of oral ATRA while confirmatory diagnostics are expedited. Regarding patients with high-risk disease, this study supports the adoption of ATRA–ATO with 2 doses of idarubicin as a new standard of care that offers better outcomes with only 5 cycles of therapy as well as a reduction in chances of differentiation syndrome, lower relapse rates, and a presumed lower risk for late anthracycline toxicities.

27. MYELOMA

Doubling Down on Bispecific Antibody Therapy for Myeloma[2]

Combined treatment with talquetamab plus teclistamab provided durable responses in patients with relapsed and refractory disease, albeit with high rates of infection. T-cell–engaging bispecific antibodies are approved as single-agent therapy for patients with relapsed myeloma who have received at least four prior lines of therapy including immunomodulatory agents, proteasome inhibitors, and an anti-CD38 monoclonal antibody. To assess the clinical utility of combining two bispecific agents with different myeloma cell antigenic targets, investigators conducted a multicenter, phase 1b–2 trial of talquetamab (anti-CD3 x anti-GPRC5D) plus teclistamab (anti-CD3 x anti-BCMA) in patients with relapsed or refractory myeloma.

Following the dose-escalation phase and utilizing a stepped-up dosing schedule to mitigate severe cytokine release syndrome (CRS), the investigators selected phase 2 doses of 0.8 mg/kg of subcutaneous talquetamab plus 3.0 mg/kg of teclistamab given with premedications on the same day every two weeks. Responding patients could be transitioned to 4-week dosing intervals. Most patients had undergone prior stem cell transplantation, and several had received prior chimeric antigen receptor T-cell or bispecific antibody therapy.

Among the 94 patients treated across all dose levels, the response rate was 76%. Serious infections occurred in 64% of patients; 11 were fatal. COVID-19 infection arose in 38 patients, with 2 deaths. Eighty-seven patients (93%) required dose modifications or delays due to adverse events, which were mostly infections; 16% discontinued one or both agents. CRS occurred in 79% of patients, almost all grade 1–2. Immune effector cell–associated neurotoxicity syndrome (ICANS) arose in only 3 patients. Among the 44 patients treated at the phase 2 dose level, the overall response rate was 80%, 52% had a complete response or better, and 86% had an ongoing response at 18 months.

This dual-targeting bispecific antibody regimen provided ongoing responses across all dose levels in very heavily pretreated patients. Encouraging responses were observed in patients with poor-risk biomarkers and extramedullary disease. CRS was well managed, but infection rates were higher than reported with single-agent bispecific therapy.

Delaying Progression from Smoldering to Active Multiple Myeloma[9]

Patients with high-risk smouldering myeloma had improved outcomes with daratumumab therapy versus active monitoring without treatment.

Smouldering myeloma, defined as monoclonal protein ≥3g/L, urine paraprotein ≥500 mg/24 hours, and/or marrow plasmacytosis of 10%–59% in the absence of myeloma-defining events, has a variable time course to progression to overt myeloma and initiation of therapy.

In a multicenter, phase 3 AQUILA trial, 390 patients with smouldering myeloma at high risk for progression to active myeloma were randomized to subcutaneous daratumumab (1800 mg subcutaneously for 39 cycles, 36 months, or until progression) or scheduled monitoring without therapy. (Daratumumab is an anti-CD38 monoclonal antibody approved for treatment of active multiple myeloma).

During a median 65-months' follow-up, the daratumumab group had a significantly lower risk of progression or death relative to the monitoring group (hazard ratio, 0.49). At 5 years, rates of progression-free survival (PFS), the primary endpoint, were 63% and 41%, respectively. Five-year overall survival also was better with daratumumab (93% vs. 87%). Serious adverse events occurred in 29% with daratumumab and 19% with monitoring; grade 3–4 infections were higher with daratumumab (16.1% vs. 4.6%). Patient-reported outcomes were similar in the two groups.

Smouldering myeloma, as defined by International Myeloma Working Group criteria, progresses to overt myeloma and related complications in a relatively short time when higher-risk features are present. The duration of follow-up in this study confirmed a significant PFS benefit with time-limited, single-agent daratumumab immunotherapy, as well as a trend toward improved overall survival, and supported its use in high-risk smouldering myeloma. Further follow-up regarding response to subsequent daratumumab-based therapy, results of additional ongoing trials that aim to delay progression in patients at high-risk, and the therapeutic benefit for Black patients (who were underrepresented in the AQUILA trial), will inform approaches to prevention of myeloma-related complications and improved survival.

Is Relapsed/Refractory Myeloma Curable?[44,86]

Possibly: 5 years after treatment with the CAR-T cell therapy ciltacabtagene autoleucel, 33% of heavily pretreated patients remained in remission.

CAR-T cell therapeutics represent a major advance for patients with relapsed/refractory and high-risk myeloma, but longer-term outcomes have been uncertain. Now, at a median follow-up of 61 months, investigators reported efficacy and safety in 97 heavily pretreated patients who received a single infusion of ciltacabtagene autoleucel (cilta-cel) in the CARTITUDE-1 trial.

Findings:

- One third of patients remain progression free.
- Durable responses occurred in patients with aberrant TP53 and high-risk cytogenetics.
- Twelve patients who achieved negative PET/CT also had undetectable minimal residual disease (MRD) after cilta-cel; all 12 remained negative on subsequent serial monitoring.

No new safety concerns were identified.

The durable remissions (including MRD negativity in the subset of patients who were tested) seen here at 5 years raise the likelihood that these patients are cured. Outcomes were better in those with lower tumor burden at initiation of CAR-T therapy. Early results in patients with relapsed myeloma point toward better progression-free survival with cilta-cel than with standard combination therapy (CARTITUDE-4 trial). Some clinicians recommend CAR-T for eligible patients as second- or third-line therapy.

Myeloma Therapy Driven by Measurable Residual Disease: De-Escalating Treatment Intensity[90]

Patients with newly diagnosed myeloma who achieved deep response after induction therapy did not benefit from high-dose chemotherapy and autologous stem cell transplantation.

Standard frontline myeloma therapy includes autologous stem cell transplant (ASCT) consolidation for medically fit patients. To test whether those who achieve deep response to induction therapy can forego ASCT, investigators conducted a phase 3 trial in patients aged 65 or younger with newly diagnosed myeloma who received 6 cycles of the quadruplet induction regimen Isa-KRd (isatuximab, carfilzomib, lenalidomide, and dexamethasone). Patients who achieved negativity of measurable residual disease (MRD) at <10^{-5} sensitivity (determined with next-generation sequencing) were randomized to ASCT plus 2 cycles of Isa-KRd versus 6 additional cycles of Isa-KRd. Patients who were MRD-positive at 10-5 sensitivity proceeded to tandem ASCT versus single ASCT plus Isa-KRd for 2 cycles.

Among the 485 patients who were MRD-negative after induction therapy, ASCT conferred no benefit over continuing Isa-KRd alone in achieving deeper response (MRD-negative at <10^{-6} sensitivity; 86% and 84%, respectively [the primary endpoint]). Of the 233 patients who remained MRD-positive after induction therapy, 32% of the tandem-ASCT group became MRD-negative before maintenance therapy compared with 40% of the single-ASCT group, a nonsignificant difference.

These results support the value of risk-adapted therapy based on postinduction MRD status, thereby permitting de-escalation of ASCT consolidation. Follow-up thus far is only 16 months, so longer-term results will be needed in order to assess durability of MRD-negative responses, progression-free survival, and, ideally, overall survival before adopting this approach in routine clinical practice.

28. MYELOFIBROSIS

Clearance of Driver Mutations after Allogeneic HSC Transplantation for Myelofibrosis[24]

In patients with myelofibrosis, clearance of driver mutations at day 30 after allogeneic HSCT appeared to influence relapse and survival, irrespective of the underlying driver mutation.

Allogeneic hematopoietic stem cell transplantation (HSCT) is the only curative treatment for myelofibrosis. Driver mutations are the pathophysiological hallmark of the disease, but the role of mutation clearance after transplantation is unclear.

In this study, the investigators used highly sensitive polymerase-chain-reaction technology to analyze the dynamics of driver mutations in peripheral-blood samples from 324 patients with myelofibrosis (73% with JAK2 mutations, 23% with CALR mutations, and 4% with MPL mutations) who were undergoing transplantation after reduced-intensity conditioning. Mutations were detected before transplantation and at 30, 100, and 180 days after transplantation to measure clearance and its effect on relapse and cure. The two primary end points were relapse and disease-free survival.

At day 30 after transplantation, mutation clearance was found in 42% of the patients who had JAK2 mutations, 73% of those who had CALR mutations, and 54% of those who had MPL mutations; the corresponding percentages at day 100 were 63%, 82%, and 100%. The cumulative incidence of relapse at 1 year was 6% (95% confidence interval [CI], 2 to 10) among patients with mutation clearance at day 30 after transplantation and 21% (95% CI, 15 to 27) among those without mutation clearance at day 30. Disease-free and overall survival at 6 years were 61% and 74%, respectively, among patients with mutation clearance at day 30 after transplantation and 41% and 60%, respectively, among those without mutation clearance at day 30. Mutation clearance at day 30 appeared to outperform traditional donor chimerism as a measure of response; it was independently associated with a reduced risk of relapse or progression (hazard ratio, 0.36; 95% CI, 0.21 to 0.61) and appeared to overcome differences in prognosis based on the type of driver mutation (JAK2 vs. MPL or CALR).

OTHER DEVELOPMENTS IN CANCER MEDICINE

29. RSV Vaccination in Stem-Cell Transplant Recipients[154]

Approximately one third of this vulnerable population had an immune response to a dose of adjuvant RSV vaccine.

Hematopoietic stem-cell transplant (HSCT) recipients are at increased risk for severe disease following infection with respiratory syncytial virus (RSV). However, limited data are available on the immunogenicity, safety, and efficacy of RSV vaccines in this population. To address this gap, researchers evaluated 94 adult HSCT recipients who received the adjuvant RSV vaccine at least 3 months posttransplant; 70% were more than 6 months posttransplant. The primary end point was sero-response, defined as at least a fourfold rise in anti–RSV pre-F protein at 4 weeks postvaccination.

Results were as follows:

- Sero-response occurred in 32% of participants. Response levels increased with longer time since transplant.
- Cell-mediated immune (CMI) responses occurred in 37% of participants.
- The most common adverse event was injection-site pain.

During a median 13 months of follow-up, RSV infection occurred in 9 participants, only 1 of whom had a humoral or CMI response to the vaccine. Two patients required intensive care unit admission.

Immune response to RSV vaccination is nearly universal in immunocompetent people. These data highlight the need for exploration of alternate vaccination strategies in HSCT recipients. However, they also demonstrate that the vaccines are safe and can generate an immune response in a modest, yet substantial, fraction of this vulnerable population. Thus, HSCT recipients should be vaccinated for RSV preferably at the onset of the RSV season, and nonpharmacologic RSV-prevention measures such as masking, hand hygiene, and social distancing at the height of the season should be maintained.

30. Anticoagulation in Patients with Cancer-Associated Pulmonary Embolism: How Long Is Long Enough?[80]

Among patients with low-risk pulmonary embolism, 18 months of anticoagulation significantly reduced its recurrence, compared with 6 months of treatment.

Cancer is a well-known risk factor for incident and recurrent venous thromboembolism (VTE), including pulmonary embolism (PE). However, the optimal duration of anticoagulation in patients with cancer and low-risk PE is unknown. In an open-label, multicenter, manufacturer-supported trial in Japan (NCT04724460), investigators randomized 179 patients with cancer-associated acute PE to 6 or 18 months of anticoagulation with rivaroxaban.

According to the simplified Pulmonary Embolism Severity Index, participants were low risk (other than cancer); 88% had incidental PE. Despite the study's premature termination due to slow recruitment, the primary outcome of recurrent VTE at 18 months occurred significantly less frequently with 18 than with 6 months of treatment (5.6% vs. 19.1%; odds ratio, 0.25). The 18-month and 6-month treatment groups did not differ significantly in the incidence of major bleeding (7.8% and 5.6%, respectively), and no fatal bleeding events occurred.

This evidence is useful for clinicians and patients who are deciding between a short and an extended duration of anticoagulation in cancer-associated VTE. Even in this prematurely terminated trial of patients with cancer, limited comorbidities, and mostly incidental PE (a feature of lower risk for recurrence), continued anticoagulation was overwhelmingly superior to short-term anticoagulation.

31. Apixaban for Extended Treatment of Provoked Venous Thromboembolism[68]

The appropriate duration of anticoagulation for venous thromboembolism (VTE) in patients who have a transient provoking factor (e.g., surgery, trauma, or immobility) and concomitant enduring risk factors is uncertain.

In this single-center, double-blind, randomized trial, adults with VTE after the occurrence of a transient provoking factor who had at least one enduring risk factor and had completed at least 3 months of anticoagulation were assigned to receive oral apixaban (at a dose of 2.5 mg twice daily) or placebo for 12 months. The primary efficacy outcome was the first symptomatic recurrent VTE. The primary safety outcome was the first episode of major bleeding.

A total of 600 patients underwent randomization (mean age, 59.5 years; female sex, 57.0%; non-White race, 19.2%). The trial population had a broad range of provoking factors and enduring risk factors. Symptomatic recurrent VTE occurred in 4 of the 300 patients (1.3%) in the apixaban group and in 30 of the 300 patients (10.0%) in the placebo group (hazard ratio, 0.13; 95% confidence interval [CI], 0.04 to 0.36; $P<0.001$). Major bleeding occurred in 1 patient in the apixaban group and none in the placebo group. Clinically relevant nonmajor bleeding was observed in 14 of 294 patients (4.8%) in the apixaban group and in 5 of 294 patients (1.7%) in the placebo group (hazard ratio, 2.68; 95% CI, 0.96 to 7.43; $P=0.06$). One patient in the apixaban group and 3 patients in the placebo group died, with no deaths attributed to cardiovascular or hemorrhagic causes. Nonhemorrhagic, nonfatal adverse events occurred in 6 patients (2.0%) in each group.

Among patients with provoked VTE and enduring risk factors, low-intensity therapy with apixaban for 12 months resulted in a lower risk of symptomatic recurrent VTE than placebo, with a low risk of major bleeding.

32. Anticoagulation and Intracranial Hemorrhage in Patients with Brain Metastases[86]

In a retrospective study, patients receiving direct oral anticoagulants had similar rates of intracranial hemorrhage compared with recipients of low-molecular-weight heparin.

Patients with brain metastases present a clinical challenge because they are at increased risk for spontaneous intracranial hemorrhage (sICH) as well as venous thromboembolism (VTE). Is one class of anticoagulation a better choice than another? Can patients with a history of sICH get another chance at anticoagulation?

To address these uncertainties, investigators examined a multinational, retrospective cohort of 505 patients with metastatic brain cancer receiving either a direct oral anticoagulant (DOAC) or low-molecular-weight heparin (LMWH) for VTE or atrial fibrillation.

Patients receiving DOACs had similar 12-month cumulative incidence of sICH compared with patients receiving LMWH (≈10%), mortality (≈50%), and VTE (≈5%).

In a multivariable analysis, patients with a history of anticoagulant-associated ICH, a bleeding disorder, concurrent aspirin use, melanoma, and renal cell carcinoma were at higher risk for ICH.

Nearly one third of patients who stopped anticoagulation resumed it within 90 days, and ICH recurred in only one patient.

DOACs are as safe as LMWH in this context and save patients from injections. However, we need to approach these patients on a case-by-case basis. The concurrent use of aspirin should be stopped unless there is a strong independent indication, and extreme caution is appropriate in starting anticoagulation in patients with melanoma or renal cell carcinoma who have brain metastases.with higher risks from the higher-dose medical-imaging tests such as CT.

33. Medical Imaging and Risk for Blood Cancers in Children and Adolescents[128]

Ionizing radiation from pediatric imaging is associated with a small but measurable, dose-dependent rise in hematologic cancer risk.

Radiation exposure from imaging studies, primarily computed tomography (CT), is a recognized risk factor for hematologic malignancy. To examine the relation between cumulative radiation exposure and risk for subsequent hematologic cancer, researchers retrospectively examined data on 3.7 million children and adolescents (a total of 35 million person-years) through age 21.

The researchers calculated radiation exposures from radiographs, fluoroscopy, angiography, nuclear medicine, and CT. Only cancer diagnoses that lagged exposure by at least 6 months were included, to avoid concerns that undiagnosed cancers had prompted the imaging. For reference, bone marrow doses of radiation for common studies vary by age of the child, but the averages are 0.02 mGy for chest x-rays, 3.8 mGy for abdominal CTs, and 13.7 mGy for head CTs.

Nearly 3,000 hematologic cancers were diagnosed. More than 7% of all children and 9% of those with hematologic cancers had received at least 1 mGy of cumulative radiation dose. Risks for hematologic malignancy increased with greater cumulative radiation doses. Compared with no exposure, patients' risk for hematologic malignancy was 1.4-fold higher with exposure of 1 to 5 mGy, 1.8-fold higher with exposure of 15 to 20 mGy, and 3.6-fold higher with exposure of 50 to 100 mGy. Translated to population-wide risks, exposures of ≥30 mGy were associated with 26 excess cancers by age 21 per 10,000 children.

Imaging remains indispensable for care of pediatric patients, but we need to use ionizing studies judiciously and apply pediatric dose-reduction protocols strictly. families.

34. A Pathway to Immunotherapeutic Targeting of Multiple Cancer Types[147]

The anti-HER2/HER3 monoclonal antibody zenocutuzumab showed activity in advanced solid tumors containing neuroregulin 1 (NRG1) gene fusions.

Neuroregulin 1 (NRG1) is an epidermal growth factor that is pathogenically altered in about 1% of solid tumors via fusion with one of many partner genes, resulting in a chimeric protein that drives oncogenesis via the HER2/HER3 pathway. These investigators conducted a multicenter, phase 2 trial of zenocutuzumab (Zeno), a bispecific anti-HER2 and anti-HER3 monoclonal antibody, in patients with advanced or metastatic cancer and an NRG1 gene fusion as detected by next-generation DNA or RNA sequencing. Eligible patients had either received prior standard therapy, which could include prior anti-HER2 antibodies or inhibitors, or were not candidates for standard therapy. Zeno infusions were administered intravenously once every 2 weeks until progression, death, or unacceptable toxicity.

Ten different tumor types were represented in the primary efficacy population (n=158). Overall, 47 patients (30%) had a treatment response, including one complete response. Response rates were 29% among the 93 patients with non–small-cell lung cancer (NSCLC) and 42% among the 36 patients with pancreatic cancer; median durations of response were 12.7 and 7.4 months, respectively. Responses also occurred in cholangiocarcinoma as well as in breast, ovarian, and gastric cancers and were observed across NRG1 fusion partners. Of the 204 patients treated with Zeno, only one discontinued because of toxicity (grade 2 pneumonitis). Grade 3 or 4 toxicities occurred infrequently; 14% of patients had grade 1 or 2 infusion reactions.

Zeno therapy was well tolerated and led to response in a subset of tumors with NRG1 fusions. These fusion mutations are best detected by RNA-based sequencing, which could be considered as a precision-medicine approach in the absence of other targetable driver mutations on standard molecular testing should Zeno move forward to regulatory approval.

35. How to Prevent Chemotherapy-Induced Peripheral Neuropathy[138]

Two low-cost interventions — hand cryotherapy and compression — reduced the incidence of neuropathy in patients treated with taxanes for early-stage breast cancer.

Chemotherapy-induced peripheral neuropathy (CIPN) is common with taxanes, platinums, vinca alkaloids, and eribulin and leads to long-term disability in up to 30% of patients. Evaluation of strategies to prevent or mitigate peripheral neuropathy has been challenging due to different methods for assessing CIPN and other conditions that can also cause peripheral neuropathy (e.g., diabetes, alcohol)

Investigators in Germany assessed the effect of hand cryotherapy and hand compression on taxane-induced peripheral neuropathy in 101 patients with early-stage breast cancer who received weekly paclitaxel or nab-paclitaxel as a component of adjuvant therapy. Patients were randomized to wear a frozen glove or two tight-fitting surgical gloves on the dominant hand 30 minutes before, during, and after treatment. The other hand served as a control. Patients with pre-existing peripheral neuropathy, prior chemotherapy, use of drugs that mask neuropathy, or certain disorders (for example, diabetes) were excluded.

Both interventions decreased the incidence of grade ≥2 CIPN — the primary outcome — but cooling had a greater effect than compression (relative risk reduction, 42% vs. 38%). With cooling, the incidence was 29% versus 50% for the control hand; with compression, 24% versus 38%. A total of 24 patients discontinued therapy, most (67%) because of CIPN. Patients experiencing grade ≥2 CIPN had reduced quality of life 6 to 8 months after completing taxane therapy compared with patients without CIPN.

Although both of this study's low-cost, easily accessible interventions effectively reduced the risk of high-grade CIPN, most clinicians will consider hand cooling easier and more patient friendly than hand constriction.

36. GLP-1 Receptor Agonist Use and Cancer Risk[142]

Data point to higher risk for some cancers and lower risk for others with GLP-1 use.

Glucagon-like peptide-1 (GLP-1) receptor agonists have been linked to excess risk for some cancers (for example, the U.S. FDA labels for these drugs note possible excess risk for thyroid cancer). However, weight loss with these drugs could lower risk for obesity-related cancers. (Obesity-related cancers are breast, thyroid, endometrial, ovarian, kidney, and colorectal cancers).Three large observational studies provide more data.

In a U.S. study of patients with obesity, overall incidence of obesity-related cancer was lower in patients who received GLP-1 agonists than in those who didn't (14 vs. 16 cancers per 1000 person-years). Risk was lower for endometrial and ovarian cancers and meningiomas, but kidney cancer was more common in GLP-1 recipients.

In a 15-year U.S. study of older patients with type 2 diabetes, obesity-related cancer incidence was similar in patients prescribed GLP-1 agonists (without metformin) and in those prescribed metformin (without GLP-1 agonists). The only cancer-specific risk difference was a higher likelihood of kidney cancer with GLP-1 use.

In a 10-year Danish study of patients with type 2 diabetes, risk for cancer was 4 percentage points higher among users of GLP-1 agonists than among users of dipeptidyl peptidase-4 inhibitors (25% vs. 21%). The only cancer-specific risk difference was a heightened incidence of uterine cancer in GLP-1 recipients.

The lower incidence of obesity-associated cancers in obese patients in the first study was remarkable. However, this finding was not observed in the two studies that focused on patients with diabetes. More troubling, in the Danish study, researchers examined all cancers (not just obesity-related cancers) and found higher risks with GLP-1 use. None of the studies showed excess risk for thyroid cancer, but the higher risk for renal cancer in two studies is of concern.

37. Overall Cancer Risk after HPV Vaccination[105]

The HPV-vaccination group had significantly fewer cancers than the control group overall (399 vs. 1090, respectively). Researchers also observed risk reductions in cancer at sites with well-established links to HPV (genitourinary and oropharyngeal), as well as other sites (gastrointestinal, respiratory, skin, hematologic, and brain).

Causal evidence demonstrates human papillomavirus (HPV) vaccination significantly reduces cervical cancer risk, and additional observational evidence supports protection of other HPV-related sites, such as genitourinary and oropharyngeal systems. To further investigate associations with noncervical cancers, researchers used a U.S.A. electronic health records database to retrospectively match 350,000 HPV-vaccinated females to controls who were not vaccinated against HPV.

- In the 5-year follow-up, the HPV-vaccination group had significantly fewer cancers than the control group overall (399 vs. 1090, respectively).
- Researchers observed risk reductions in cancer at sites with well-established links to HPV (genitourinary and oropharyngeal), as well as other sites (gastrointestinal, respiratory, skin, hematologic, and brain).
- Vaccination at 9–14 years conferred better protection than at 15–26 years, with the 9-valent HPV formulation providing greater benefit than the 4-valent formulation in most categories.

These data are interesting but should be viewed with caution since the observed cancer reduction include different cancer types, including sites not known to be linked to HPV. However, this large dataset reinforces the idea that earlier and complete vaccination beginning at 9 years provides the best possible protection against HPV-related cancers.

38. Covid-19 mRNA Vaccines Aid Immune Checkpoint Inhibitor Cancer Therapy[110]

Receiving a vaccine that is not directed at tumor antigens can improve survival.

Many cancers elicit T-cell attacks. But these cancer cells also produce “checkpoint” molecules on their surface that attach to receptors on the attacking T cells. This “handshake” between the cancer cells and the T cells allows the cancer to grow. Previously, researchers had shown that immune checkpoint inhibitors (ICIs) can improve the T cell attack dramatically and can improve the patient’s outcome. However, ICIs do not work in all types of cancer.

Previous studies in animals showed that SARS-CoV-2 (Covid-19) mRNA vaccines prime the attacking CD8+ T cells and augment the effect of ICI drugs. In an observational study of patients who received ICI therapy, investigators compared outcomes among patients who received the mRNA vaccines within 100 days of starting ICI therapy and those who did not.

- In 1000 patients with unresectable stage III or stage IV non–small-cell lung cancer and in 200 patients with stage IV melanoma, median and 3-year overall survival were significantly better in those who had received mRNA vaccines near the start of ICI therapy.
- In both animal and preclinical human studies, the researchers showed that the mRNA vaccines augmented the immune response by increasing production of type I interferon, which activated myeloid cells and lymphocytes.

The authors suggested that activating the innate immune system with a vaccine (such as the Covid-19 mRNA vaccine, which is not directed at tumor antigens) near the start of immune checkpoint inhibitor (ICI) therapy might improve survival greatly, at least for patients with one of these two end-stage cancers.

39. Caring for Long-Term Survivors of Childhood Cancer[83]

Late-onset treatment-related complications led to higher mortality; care providers should prioritize monitoring and management of cancer survivors.

The dramatic progress in curing childhood and adolescent/young adult malignancies has been tempered by lethal treatment-related cancers and cardiovascular complications. In a retrospective multicenter study, investigators compared mortality rates in childhood/young adolescents and young adult cancer survivors diagnosed before age 21 who survived to or beyond age 50 against rates in the general population, and compared chronic health conditions in a cohort of consenting survivors and their siblings.

Among 7490 survivors, mortality risks after age 50 were 8.6% at 5 years, 18.4% at 10 years, and 32.7% at 15 years, exceeding the risk in the general population. The greatest excess mortality was observed among Hodgkin's lymphoma survivors.

Cancer, most commonly respiratory, was the primary cause of death among survivors and was strongly related to prior radiation therapy. Survivors had two to three times higher rates of high-grade chronic health conditions than their siblings. Prior radiation therapy conferred significant risk, but not prior chemotherapy.

Oncologists and primary care providers should educate their patients about the importance of cancer screening, lifelong health monitoring, and the management of chronic conditions, including cardiovascular risk factors and diseases. While this is especially true for those treated with radiotherapy, the impact of previous chemotherapy may have been underrepresented in this study as complications typically arise within 10 to 20 years after initial treatment.

40. CONCLUSIONS

Of the four most common cancers, breast cancer had the largest number of new reports with 26. Colo-rectal cancer was second with 18 reports, followed by non-small cell lung cancer with 11 and prostate cancer with 7. There were 7 new reports on non-Hodgkin lymphoma. The field continues to develop at an exponential rate

41. REFERENCES

1. Chibaudel B et al. Assessment of the addition of oxaliplatin to fluoropyrimidine-based adjuvant chemotherapy in patients with high-risk stage II colon cancer: An ACCENT pooled analysis. J Clin Oncol 2024 Dec 10; 42:4187. (https://doi.org/10.1200/JCO.24.00394)

2. Cohen YC et al. Talquetamab plus teclistamab in relapsed or refractory multiple myeloma. N Engl J Med 2025 Jan 9; 392:138. (https://doi.org/10.1056/NEJMoa2406536)

3. Shubeck SP, Morrow M, Dossett LA. De-escalation in breast cancer surgery. NPJ Breast Cancer. 2022 Feb 23;8(1):25. doi: 10.1038/s41523-022-00383-4. PMID: 35197478; PMCID: PMC8866473.

4. Harborg S, et al. Postdiagnosis statin use and breast cancer mortality. JAMA Netw Open 2025 Oct 1; 8:e2538737. DOI: 10.1001/jamanetworkopen.2025.38737.

5. Reimer T et al. Axillary surgery in breast cancer — Primary results of the INSEMA trial. N Engl J Med 2024 Dec 12; [e-pub]. (https://doi.org/10.1056/NEJMoa2412063)

6. Ghobadi A et al. Induced pluripotent stem-cell-derived CD19-directed chimeric antigen receptor natural killer cells in B-cell lymphoma: A phase 1, first-in-human trial. Lancet 2025 Jan 11; 405:127. (https://doi.org/10.1016/S0140-6736(24)02462-0)

7. Shapiro RM and Romee R. iPSC-derived CD19 CAR NK cells for relapsed or refractory lymphoma. Lancet 2025 Jan 11; 405:98. (https://doi.org/10.1016/S0140-6736(24)02524-8)

8. Heger J-M et al. Circulating tumor DNA sequencing for biologic classification and individualized risk stratification in patients with Hodgkin lymphoma. J Clin Oncol 2024 Dec 10; 42:4218. (https://doi.org/10.1200/JCO.23.01867)

9. Dimopoulos MA et al. Daratumumab or active monitoring for high-risk smoldering multiple myeloma. N Engl J Med 2024 Dec 9; [e-pub]. (https://doi.org/10.1056/NEJMoa2409029)

10. Randon G et al. Ramucirumab plus paclitaxel as switch maintenance versus continuation of first-line oxaliplatin-based chemotherapy in patients with advanced HER2-negative gastric or gastro-oesophageal junction cancer (ARMANI): A randomised, open-label, multicentre, phase 3 trial. Lancet Oncol 2024 Dec; 25:1539. (https://doi.org/10.1016/S1470-2045(24)00580-1)

11. Jhaveri KL et al. Imlunestrant with or without abemaciclib in advanced breast cancer. N Engl J Med 2024 Dec 11; [e-pub]. (https://doi.org/10.1056/NEJMoa2410858)

12. Andre T et al. Nivolumab plus ipilimumab in microsatellite-instability–high metastatic colorectal cancer. N Engl J Med 2024 Nov 28; 391:2014. (https://doi.org/10.1056/NEJMoa2402141)

13. Langerbeins P et al. Ibrutinib in early-stage chronic lymphocytic leukemia: The randomized, placebo-controlled, double-blind, phase III CLL12 trial. J Clin Oncol 2024 Nov 27; [e-pub]. (https://doi.org/10.1200/JCO.24.00975)

14. Pavlakis N et al. INTEGRATE IIa phase III study: Regorafenib for refractory advanced gastric cancer. J Clin Oncol 2024 Oct 4; [e-pub]. (https://doi.org/10.1200/JCO.24.00055)

15. Roddie C et al. Obecabtagene autoleucel in adults with B-cell acute lymphoblastic leukemia. N Engl J Med 2024 Nov 27; 391:2219. (https://doi.org/10.1056/NEJMoa2406526)

16. Bossi A et al. Efficacy and safety of prostate radiotherapy in de novo metastatic castration-sensitive prostate cancer (PEACE-1): A multicentre, open-label, randomised, phase 3 study with a 2 x 2 factorial design. Lancet 2024 Nov 23; 404:2065. (https://doi.org/10.1016/S0140-6736(24)01865-8)

17. Turner NC et al. Inavolisib-based therapy in PIK3CA-mutated advanced breast cancer. N Engl J Med 2024 Oct 31; 391:1584. (https://doi.org/10.1056/NEJMoa2404625)

18. Yamashita Y et al. Rivaroxaban for 18 months versus 6 months in patients with cancer and acute low-risk pulmonary embolism: An open-label, multicenter, randomized clinical trial (ONCO PE Trial). Circulation 2024 Nov 18; [e-pub]. (https://doi.org/10.1161/CIRCULATIONAHA.124.072758)

19. Adam R et al. Liver transplantation plus chemotherapy versus chemotherapy alone in patients with permanently unresectable colorectal liver metastases (TransMet): Results from a multicentre, open-label, prospective, randomised controlled trial. Lancet 2024 Sep 21; 404:1107. (https://doi.org/10.1016/S0140-6736(24)01595-2)

20. Tedeschi A et al. Atezolizumab, venetoclax, and obinutuzumab combination in Richter transformation diffuse large B-cell lymphoma (MOLTO): A multicentre, single-arm, phase 2 trial. Lancet Oncol 2024 Oct; 25:1298. (https://doi.org/10.1016/S1470-2045(24)00396-6)

21. Hoeppner J et al. Perioperative chemotherapy or preoperative chemoradiotherapy in esophageal cancer. N Engl J Med 2025 Jan 23; 392:323. (https://doi.org/10.1056/NEJMoa2409408)

22. Fakih MG et al. Sotorasib plus panitumumab in refractory colorectal cancer with mutated KRAS G12C. N Engl J Med 2023 Oct 22; [e-pub]. (https://doi.org/10.1056/NEJMoa2308795)

23. Geyer, CE et al. Survival with Trastuzumab Emtansine in Residual HER2-Positive Breast Cancer. N Engl J Med 2025;392:249-257. DOI: 10.1056/NEJMoa2406070

24. Gagelmann, N et al. Clearance of Driver Mutations after Transplantation for Myelofibrosis. N Engl J Med 2025;392:150-160. DOI: 10.1056/NEJMoa2408941

25. Apolo, AB et al. Adjuvant Pembrolizumab versus Observation in Muscle-Invasive Urothelial Carcinoma. N Engl J Med 2025;392:45-55. DOI: 10.1056/NEJMoa2401726

26. Wolchok, JD et al. Final, 10-Year Outcomes with Nivolumab plus Ipilimumab in Advanced Melanoma. N Engl J Med 2025;392:11-22. DOI: 10.1056/NEJMoa2407417

27. Hwang ES et al. Active monitoring with or without endocrine therapy for low-risk ductal carcinoma in situ: The COMET randomized clinical trial. JAMA 2024 Dec 12; [e-pub]. (https://doi.org/10.1001/jama.2024.26698)

28. Jain MD et al. Five-year follow-up of standard-of-care axicabtagene ciloleucel for large B-cell lymphoma: Results from the US Lymphoma CAR T Consortium. J Clin Oncol 2024 Oct 20; 42:3581. (https://doi.org/10.1200/JCO.23.02786)

29. Potluri VS et al. The association of Epstein–Barr virus donor and recipient serostatus with outcomes after kidney transplantation: A retrospective cohort study. Ann Intern Med 2025 Jan 28; [e-pub]. (https://doi.org/10.7326/ANNALS-24-00165

30. Dorali P et al. Cervical cancer mortality among US women younger than 25 years, 1992–2021. JAMA 2025 Jan 14; 333:165. (https://doi.org/10.1001/jama.2024.22169)

31. Zhang X et al. First-line sugemalimab plus chemotherapy for advanced gastric cancer: The GEMSTONE-303 randomized clinical trial. JAMA 2025 Feb 24; [e-pub]. (https://doi.org/10.1001/jama.2024.28463)

32. Jillella AP et al. Academic community partnership in acute promyelocytic leukemia and early mortality: The ECOG-ACRIN EA9131 trial. JAMA Oncol 2025 Feb 27; [e-pub]. (https://doi.org/10.1001/jamaoncol.2024.7033)

33. Guarneri V, Lenihan DJ, Valero V, Durand JB, Broglio K, Hess KR, Michaud LB, Gonzalez-Angulo AM, Hortobagyi GN, Esteva FJ. Long-term cardiac tolerability of trastuzumab in metastatic breast cancer: the M.D. Anderson Cancer Center experience. J Clin Oncol. 2006 Sep 1;24(25):4107-15. doi: 10.1200/JCO.2005.04.9551. Epub 2006 Aug 14. Erratum in: J Clin Oncol. 2008 May 10;26(14): 2421. PMID: 16908934.

34. van der Lei S et al. Thermal ablation versus surgical resection of small-size colorectal liver metastases (COLLISION): An international, randomised, controlled, phase 3 non-inferiority trial. Lancet Oncol 2025 Feb; 26:187. (https://doi.org/10.1016/S1470-2045(24)00660-0)

35. Ignatiadis M et al. Adjuvant atezolizumab for early triple-negative breast cancer: The ALEXANDRA/IMpassion030 randomized clinical trial. JAMA 2025 Jan 30; [e-pub]. (https://doi.org/10.1001/jama.2024.26886)

36. Shroff RT et al. SWOG S1815: A phase III randomized trial of gemcitabine, cisplatin, and nab-paclitaxel versus gemcitabine and cisplatin in newly diagnosed, advanced biliary tract cancers. J Clin Oncol 2025 Feb 10; 43:536. (https://doi.org/10.1200/JCO-24-01383)

37. Brown JR et al. Fixed-duration acalabrutinib combinations in untreated chronic lymphocytic leukemia. N Engl J Med 2025 Feb 20; 392:748. (https://doi.org/10.1056/NEJMoa2409804)

38. André T et al. Nivolumab plus ipilimumab versus nivolumab in microsatellite instability-high metastatic colorectal cancer (CheckMate 8HW): A randomised, open-label, phase 3 trial. Lancet 2025 Feb 1; 405:383. (https://doi.org/10.1016/S0140-6736(24)02848-4)

39. Dawson LA et al. Stereotactic body radiotherapy vs sorafenib alone in hepatocellular carcinoma: The NRG Oncology/RTOG 1112 phase 3 randomized clinical trial. JAMA Oncol 2025 Feb; 11:136. (https://doi.org/10.1001/jamaoncol.2024.5403)colo

40. Kudo M et al. Transarterial chemoembolisation combined with lenvatinib plus pembrolizumab versus dual placebo for unresectable, non-metastatic hepatocellular carcinoma (LEAP-012): A multicentre, randomised, double-blind, phase 3 study. Lancet 2025 Jan 18; 405:203. (https://doi.org/10.1016/S0140-6736(24)02575-3)

41. Schram AM et al. Efficacy of zenocutuzumab in NRG1 fusion–positive cancer. N Engl J Med 2025 Feb 6; 392:566. (https://doi.org/10.1056/NEJMoa2405008)

42. Gupta, S et al. Blinatumomab in Standard-Risk B-Cell Acute Lymphoblastic Leukemia in Children. N Engl J Med 2025;392:875-891. DOI: 10.1056/NEJMoa2411680

43. Chan, JA. Phase 3 Trial of Cabozantinib to Treat Advanced Neuroendocrine Tumors. N Engl J Med 2025; 392:653-665. DOI: 10.1056/NEJMoa2403991

44. Harrison, SJ et al. CAR+ T-Cell Lymphoma after Cilta-cel Therapy for Relapsed or Refractory Myeloma. N Engl J Med 2025;392:677-685DOI: 10.1056/NEJMoa2309728

45. Perica, P et al. CD4+ T-Cell Lymphoma Harboring a Chimeric Antigen Receptor Integration in TP53. N Engl J Med 2025;392:577-583. DOI: 10.1056/NEJMoa2411507

46. Kopetz S et al. Encorafenib, cetuximab and chemotherapy in BRAF-mutant colorectal cancer: A randomized phase 3 trial. Nat Med 2025 Mar; 31:901. (https://doi.org/10.1038/s41591-024-03443-3)

47. Machtay M et al. Postoperative radiotherapy ± cetuximab for intermediate-risk head and neck cancer. J Clin Oncol 2025 Jan 22; [e-pub]. (https://doi.org/10.1200/JCO-24-01829)

48. Baxter SM et al. Glucagon-like peptide 1 receptor agonists and risk of thyroid cancer: An international multisite cohort study. Thyroid 2025 Jan; 35:69. (https://doi.org/10.1089/thy.2024.0387)

49. Nilson, DH. Report from the 2025 ASCO Gastrointestinal Cancers Symposium. N Engl J Med. Feb 10th 2025

50. Platzbecker U, et al. Arsenic trioxide and all-trans retinoic acid combination therapy for the treatment of high-risk acute promyelocytic leukemia: Results from the APOLLO trial. J Clin Oncol 2025 Aug 18; [e-pub]. (https://doi.org/10.1200/JCO-25-00535)

51. Iland HJ. APOLLO: Optimizing the treatment of high-risk acute promyelocytic leukemia with all-trans retinoic acid and arsenic trioxide while minimizing the role of chemotherapy. J Clin Oncol 2025 Aug 18; [e-pub]. (https://doi.org/10.1200/JCO-25-01496)

52. Minson A et al. Glofitamab combined with Pola-R-CHP or R-CHOP as first therapy in younger patients with high-risk large B-cell lymphoma: Results from the COALITION study. J Clin Oncol 2025 Aug 10; 43:2595. (https://doi.org/10.1200/JCO-25-00481)

53. van Hemert AKE et al. Iodine seed–marking protocol for response-guided axillary treatment after systemic therapy for node-positive breast cancer. JAMA Oncol 2025 Aug 28; [e-pub]. (https://doi.org/10.1001/jamaoncol.2025.2752)

54. Tarantino P et al. Outcomes of subsequent treatment regimens after trastuzumab deruxtecan in patients with metastatic breast cancer. J Natl Cancer Inst 2025 Aug 14; [e-pub]. (https://doi.org/10.1093/jnci/djaf220)

55. Ryser MD et al. Cancer outcomes in women without upfront surgery for ductal carcinoma in situ: Observational cohort study. BMJ 2025 Jul 8; 390:e083542. (https://doi.org/10.1136/bmj-2024-083542)

56. Cardoso F et al. Elinzanetant for Vasomotor Symptoms from Endocrine Therapy for Breast Cancer. NEJM, 2025/08/21, doi: 10.1056/NEJMoa2415566

57. Cascone, T et al. Perioperative Nivolumab in Resectable Lung Cancer. N Engl J Med 2024; 390:1756-1769. DOI: 10.1056/NEJMoa2311926

58. Campone, M et al. Vepdegestrant, a PROTAC Estrogen Receptor Degrader, in Advanced Breast Cancer. N Engl J Med 2025; 393:556-568. DOI: 10.1056/NEJMoa2505725

59. Reuss JE et al. Therapy for stage IV non–small cell lung cancer with driver alterations: ASCO living guideline, version 2025.1. J Clin Oncol 2025 Aug 20; 43:e31. (https://doi.org/10.1200/JCO-25-01061)

60. Owen DH et al. Therapy for stage IV non–small cell lung cancer without driver alterations: ASCO living guideline, version 2025.1. J Clin Oncol 2025 Aug 20;43:e45. (https://doi.org/10.1200/JCO-25-01062)

61. Suzuki Y et al. Survival after fertility-preserving hormonal therapy vs hysterectomy for early-stage endometrial cancer. JAMA Oncol 2025 Aug 28; [e-pub]. (https://doi.org/10.1001/jamaoncol.2025.2761)

62. Martling A et al. Low-dose aspirin for PI3K-altered localized colorectal cancer. N Engl J Med 2025 Sep 18; 393:1051. (https://doi.org/10.1056/NEJMoa2504650)

63. Babiker HM et al. Tumor treating fields with gemcitabine and nab-paclitaxel for locally advanced pancreatic adenocarcinoma: Randomized, open-label, pivotal phase III PANOVA-3 study. J Clin Oncol 2025 Jul 20; 43:2350. (https://doi.org/10.1200/JCO-25-00746)

64. Dai H et al. GLP-1 receptor agonists and cancer risk in adults with obesity. JAMA Oncol 2025 Aug 21; [e-pub]. (https://doi.org/10.1001/jamaoncol.2025.2681)

65. Lu Y et al. Association of glucagon-like peptide-1 receptor agonists with cancer risk in older adults with type 2 diabetes. Obesity 2025 Aug 21; [e-pub]. (https://doi.org/10.1002/oby.24366)

66. Gamborg M et al. Long-term cancer risk in users ofagonists in Denmark: A nationwide et al. Lancet Res Health Eur 2025 Aug

67. Keating NL et al. Diabetes and cardiovascular disease during androgen deprivation therapy for prostate cancer. J Clin Oncol 2006 Sep 20; 24:4448-56.

68. Piazza, G et al. Apixaban for Extended Treatment of Provoked Venous Thromboembolism. N Engl J Med 2025; 393:1166-1176. DOI: 10.1056/NEJMoa2509426

69. Munir, T et al. Measurable Residual Disease–Guided Therapy for Chronic Lymphocytic Leukemia. N Engl J Med 2025; 393:1177-1190. DOI: 10.1056/NEJMoa2504341

70. Chia SB et al. Respiratory viral infections awaken metastatic breast cancer cells in lungs. Nature 2025 Jul 30; [e-pub]. (https://doi.org/10.1038/s41586-025-09332-0)

71. Ford AC et al. Eradication therapy to prevent gastric cancer in Helicobacter pylori–positive individuals: Systematic review and meta-analysis of randomized controlled trials and observational studies. Gastroenterology 2025 Aug; 169:261. (https://doi.org/10.1053/j.gastro.2024.12.033)

72. Wiklund A-K et al. Risk of gastric adenocarcinoma after eradication of Helicobacter pylori.Gastroenterology 2025 Aug; 169:244. (https://doi.org/10.1053/j.gastro.2025.01.239)

73. Shah SC et al. AGA clinical practice update on screening and surveillance in individuals at increased risk for gastric cancer in the United States: Expert review. Gastroenterology 2025 Feb; 168:405. (https://doi.org/10.1053/j.gastro.2024.11.001)

74. Uppaluri R et al. Neoadjuvant and adjuvant pembrolizumab in locally advanced head and neck cancer. N Engl J Med 2025 Jul 3; 393:37. (https://doi.org/10.1056/NEJMoa2415434)

75. Rischin D et al. Adjuvant cemiplimab or placebo in high-risk cutaneous squamous-cell carcinoma. N Engl J Med 2025 May 31; [e-pub]. (https://doi.org/10.1056/NEJMoa2502449)

76. Courneya KS et al. Structured exercise after adjuvant chemotherapy for colon cancer. N Engl J Med 2025 Jul 3; 393:13. (https://doi.org/10.1056/NEJMoa2502760)

77. Mountzios G et al. Tarlatamab in small-cell lung cancer after platinum-based chemotherapy. N Engl J Med 2025 Jun 2; [e-pub]. (https://doi.org/10.1056/NEJMoa2502099)

78. Rao S et al. Retifanlimab with carboplatin and paclitaxel for locally recurrent or metastatic squamous cell carcinoma of the anal canal (POD1UM-303/InterAACT-2): A global, phase 3 randomised controlled trial. Lancet 2025 Jun 14; 405:2144. (https://doi.org/10.1016/S0140-6736(25)00631-2)

79. Rutherford SC et al. Nivolumab-AVD versus brentuximab vedotin–AVD in older patients with advanced-stage classic Hodgkin lymphoma enrolled on S1826. J Clin Oncol 2025 Jun 16; [e-pub]. (https://doi.org/10.1200/JCO-25-00204)

80. Mahmoud A et al. Reduced-dose versus full-dose direct oral anticoagulants for extended secondary venous thromboembolism prophylaxis in cancer patients: A systematic review and meta-analysis of randomized trials. Am J Hematol 2025 Sep 24; [e-pub]. (https://doi.org/10.1002/ajh.70090)

81. Curtis DJ et al. Graft-versus-host disease prophylaxis with cyclophosphamide and cyclosporin. N Engl J Med 2025 Jun 13; [e-pub]. (https://doi.org/10.1056/NEJMoa2503189)

82. Lötscher J et al. Respiratory syncytial virus vaccination in adult allogeneic hematopoietic cell transplant recipients. JAMA 2025 Oct 2; [e-pub]. (https://doi.org/10.1001/jama.2025.16744)

83. Bhandari R, et al. Health outcomes beyond age 50 years in survivors of childhood cancer: A report from the Childhood Cancer Survivor Study. J Clin Oncol 2025 Sep 20; 43:2998 10.1200/JCO-25-00385.40789102

84. Fitzpatrick MB et al. Clinical validation of a vaginal cervical cancer screening self-collection method for at-home use: A nonrandomized clinical trial. JAMA Netw Open 2025 May; 8:e2511081. (https://doi.org/10.1001/jamanetworkopen.2025.11081)

85. Jagannath S et al. Long-term (≥5-Year) remission and survival after treatment with ciltacabtagene autoleucel in CARTITUDE-1 patients with relapsed/refractory multiple myeloma. J Clin Oncol 2025 Jun 3; [e-pub]. (https://doi.org/10.1200/JCO-25-00760)

86. Hamulyák EN et al. Multinational cohort study of intracranial hemorrhage in patients with brain metastases receiving anticoagulation. Haematologica 2025 Jun; 110:1417. (https://doi.org/10.3324/haematol.2024.286973)

87. Yau T et al. Nivolumab plus ipilimumab versus lenvatinib or sorafenib as first-line treatment for unresectable hepatocellular carcinoma (CheckMate 9DW): An open-label, randomised, phase 3 trial. Lancet 2025 May 24; 405:1851. (https://doi.org/10.1016/S0140-6736(25)00403-9)

88. Srinivasan R et al. Bevacizumab and erlotinib in hereditary and sporadic papillary kidney cancer. N Engl J Med 2025 Jun 19; 392:2346. (https://doi.org/10.1056/NEJMoa2200900)

89. Cardoso F et al. Elinzanetant for vasomotor symptoms from endocrine therapy for breast cancer. N Engl J Med 2025 Jun 2; [e-pub]. (https://doi.org/10.1056/NEJMoa2415566)

90. Perrot A et al. Measurable residual disease–guided therapy in newly diagnosed myeloma. N Engl J Med 2025 Jun 3; [e-pub]. (https://doi.org/10.1056/NEJMoa2505133)

91. Shitara K et al. Trastuzumab deruxtecan or ramucirumab plus paclitaxel in gastric cancer. N Engl J Med 2025 May 31; [e-pub]. (https://doi.org/10.1056/NEJMoa2503119)

92. Bidard F-C et al. First-line camizestrant for emerging ESR1-mutated advanced breast cancer. N Engl J Med 2025 Jun 1; [e-pub]. (https://doi.org/10.1056/NEJMoa2502929)

93. Janjigian YY et al. Perioperative durvalumab in gastric and gastroesophageal junction cancer. N Engl J Med 2025 Jun 1; [e-pub]. (https://doi.org/10.1056/NEJMoa2503701)

94. Elez E et al. Encorafenib, cetuximab, and mFOLFOX6 in BRAF-mutated colorectal cancer. N Engl J Med 2025 May 30; [e-pub]. (https://doi.org/10.1056/NEJMoa2501912)

95. Jhaveri KL et al. Overall survival with inavolisib in PIK3CA-mutated advanced breast cancer. N Engl J Med 2025 May 31; [e-pub]. (https://doi.org/10.1056/NEJMoa2501796)

96. Blondeaux E et al. Association between risk-reducing surgeries and survival in young BRCA carriers with breast cancer: An international cohort study. Lancet Oncol 2025 Jun; 26:759. (https://doi.org/10.1016/S1470-2045(25)00152-4)

98. Cinciripini PM et al. Survival outcomes of an early intervention smoking cessation treatment after a cancer diagnosis. JAMA Oncol 2024 Dec; 10:1689. (https://doi.org/10.1001/jamaoncol.2024.4890)

99. Geyer CE Jr et al. Survival with trastuzumab emtansine in residual HER2-positive breast cancer. N Engl J Med 2025 Jan 16; 392:249. (https://doi.org/10.1056/NEJMoa2406070)

100. Vogel-Claussen J, et al. Effectiveness of NELSON versus PLCOm2012 lung cancer screening eligibility criteria in Germany (HANSE): A prospective cohort study. Lancet Oncol 2025 Dec; 26:1541 10.1016/S1470-2045(25)00490-5.41232542

101. Hadizadeh F, et al. Hormonal contraceptive formulations and breast cancer risk in adolescents and premenopausal women. JAMA Oncol 2025 Oct 30; [e-pub] 10.1001/jamaoncol.2025.4480.41165687

102. Pastorino A, et al. The definition of cure in colon cancer: A pooled analysis of 15 randomized clinical trials. JAMA Oncol 2025 Dec; 11:1440. DOI: 10.1001/jamaoncol.2025.3760.

103. Old O, et al. Barrett's Oesophagus Surveillance Versus Endoscopy at Need Study (BOSS): A Randomized Controlled Trial. Gastroenterology 2025 Nov; 169:1233. DOI: 10.1053/j.gastro.2025.03.021.

104. Attard G, et al. Niraparib and abiraterone acetate plus prednisone for HRR-deficient metastatic castration-sensitive prostate cancer: A randomized phase 3 trial. Nat Med 2025 Dec; 31:4109. DOI: 10.1038/s41591-025-03961-8.

105. Hung Y-M, et al. HPV vaccination is associated with lower risk of cancers among females. Am J Med 2025 Oct 23; [e-pub]. DOI: 10.1016/j.amjmed.2025.10.016.

106. Pickersgill NA, et al. Prostate-specific antigen levels among participants receiving annual testing. JAMA Oncol 2025 Nov; 11:1341 10.1001/jamaoncol.2025.3386.40965920

107. Hecht JR, et al. Zanzalintinib plus atezolizumab versus regorafenib in refractory colorectal cancer (STELLAR-303): A randomised, open-label, phase 3 trial. Lancet 2025 Nov 15; 406:2360 10.1016/S0140-6736(25)02025-2.41130252

108. Wang Z, et al. Perioperative camrelizumab plus rivoceranib versus surgery alone in patients with resectable hepatocellular carcinoma at intermediate or high risk of recurrence (CARES-009): A randomised phase 2/3 trial. Lancet 2025 Nov 1; 406:2089 10.1016/S0140-6736(25)01720-9.41125112

109. Kunkler IH, et al. Ten-year survival after postmastectomy chest-wall irradiation in breast cancer. N Engl J Med 2025 Nov 6; 393:1771 10.1056/NEJMoa2412225.41191939

110. Grippin AJ, et al. SARS-CoV-2 mRNA vaccines sensitize tumours to immune checkpoint blockade. Nature 2025 Oct 22; [e-pub] 10.1038/s41586-025-09655-y.41125896

111. Jimenez, CN et al. Belzutifan for Advanced Pheochromocytoma or Paraganglioma. N Engl J Med 2025;393:2012-2022. DOI: 10.1056/NEJMoa2504964

112. Le, X et al. Sevabertinib in Advanced *HER2*-Mutant Non–Small-Cell Lung Cancer. N Engl J Med 2025;393:1819-1832. DOI: 10.1056/NEJMoa2511065

113. Cortés, J et al. Sacituzumab Govitecan in Untreated, Advanced Triple-Negative Breast Cancer. N Engl J Med 2025;393:1912-1925. DOI: 10.1056/NEJMoa2511734

114. Kunkler, IH et al. Ten-Year Survival after Postmastectomy Chest-Wall Irradiation in Breast Cancer. N Engl J Med 2025;393:1771-1783. DOI: 10.1056/NEJMoa2412225

115. Jänne PA, et al. Survival with osimertinib plus chemotherapy in EGFR-mutated advanced NSCLC. N Engl J Med 2025 Oct 17; [e-pub] 10.1056/NEJMoa2510308.41104938

116. Roobol MJ, et al. European study of prostate cancer screening — 23-year follow-up. N Engl J Med 2025 Oct 30; 393:1669 10.1056/NEJMoa2503223.41160819

117. Karna R, et al. Performance of fecal immunochemical test in individuals with personal history of polyps and family history of colorectal cancer: A systematic review. Clin Gastroenterol Hepatol 2025 Sep 16; [e-pub] 10.1016/j.cgh.2025.09.013.40967445

118. Bochner E, et al. Assessing the diagnostic performance of renal ultrasound in microhematuria evaluation: Validation of the AUA microhematuria 2020 guidelines. Urology 2025 Sep 11; [e-pub] 10.1016/j.urology.2025.09.012.40946922

119. Arayakarnkul S, et al. Endoscopic submucosal dissection for previously attempted colorectal lesions: An international multicenter experience. Clin Gastroenterol Hepatol 2025 Oct; 23:1925

120. Yang, H-C et al. Overall Survival with Amivantamab–Lazertinib in EGFR-Mutated Advanced NSCLC. N Engl J Med 2025;393:1681-1693. DOI: 10.1056/NEJMoa2503001

121. Tolaney, SM et al. Trastuzumab Deruxtecan plus Pertuzumab for HER2-Positive Metastatic Breast Cancer. NEJM DOI: 10.1056/NEJMoa2508668

122. Powles, T et al. ctDNA-Guided Adjuvant Atezolizumab in Muscle-Invasive Bladder Cancer. N Engl J Med 2025;393:2395-2408. DOI: 10.1056/NEJMoa2511885

123. Sheng, X et al. Disitamab Vedotin plus Toripalimab in HER2-Expressing Advanced Urothelial Cancer. N Engl J Med 2025;393:2324-2337. DOI: 10.1056/NEJMoa2511648

124. Shore, ND et al. Improved Survival with Enzalutamide in Biochemically Recurrent Prostate Cancer. N Eng J Med. DOI: 10.1056/NEJMoa2510310

125. Fang, W et al. Sacituzumab Tirumotecan in EGFR-TKI–Resistant, EGFR-Mutated Advanced NSCL. N Engl J Med 2026;394:13-26. DOI: 10.1056/NEJMoa2512071

126. Ascierto, PA et al. Nivolumab for Resected Stage III or IV Melanoma at 9 Years. N Eng J Med. DOI: 10.1056/NEJMoa2504966

127. Tu, H et al. Sentinel-Lymph-Node Biopsy Alone or with Lymphadenectomy in Cervical Cancer. N Engl J Med 2025;393:1463-1474. DOI: 10.1056/NEJMoa2506267

128. Smith-Bindman, R et al. Medical Imaging and Pediatric and Adolescent Hematologic Cancer Risk. N Engl J Med 2025;393:1269-1278. DOI: 10.1056/NEJMoa2502098. DOI: 10.1056/NEJMoa2502114

129. Ye P et al. Resolution of Squamous-Cell Carcinoma by Restoring T-Cell Receptor Signaling. N Engl J Med 2025;393:469-478. DOI: 10.1056/NEJMoa2502114

130. Cercek, A et al. Nonoperative Management of Mismatch Repair–Deficient Tumors. N Engl J Med 2025;392:2297-2308. DOI: 10.1056/NEJMoa2404512

131. Heymach, JV et al. Zongertinib in Previously Treated HER2-Mutant Non–Small-Cell Lung Cancer. N Engl J Med 2025;392:2321-2333DOI: 10.1056/NEJMoa2503704

132. Mamounas, EP et al. Omitting Regional Nodal Irradiation after Response to Neoadjuvant Chemotherapy. N Engl J Med 2025;392:2113-2124. DOI: 10.1056/NEJMoa2414859

133. Forde, PM et al. Overall Survival with Neoadjuvant Nivolumab plus Chemotherapy in Lung Cancer. N Engl J Med 2025;393:741-752. DOI: 10.1056/NEJMoa2502931

134. Svoboda, J et al. Enhanced CAR T-Cell Therapy for Lymphoma after Previous Failure. N Engl J Med 2025;392:1, 824-1835. DOI: 10.1056/NEJMoa2408771

135. Raghav, K. Carcinoma of unknown primary site. N Engl J Med 2025;392:2035-2047. DOI: 10.1056/NEJMcp2402691

136. Foà, R. Ph-Positive Acute Lymphoblastic Leukemia — 25 Years of Progress. N Engl J Med 2025;392:1941-1952. DOI: 10.1056/NEJMra2405573

137. Gilbert FJ et al. Comparison of supplemental breast cancer imaging techniques — Interim results from the BRAID randomised controlled trial. Lancet 2025 May 31; 405:1935. (https://doi.org/10.1016/S0140-6736(25)00582-3)

138. Michel LL et al. Efficacy of hand cooling and compression in preventing taxane-induced neuropathy: The POLAR randomized clinical trial. JAMA Oncol 2025 Apr 1; 11:408. (https://doi.org/10.1001/jamaoncol.2025.0001)

139. Ye P et al. Resolution of Squamous-Cell Carcinoma by Restoring T-Cell Receptor Signaling. N Engl J Med 2025;393:469-478. DOI: 10.1056/NEJMoa2502114

140. Xie W-H et al. Four cycles of docetaxel plus cisplatin as neoadjuvant chemotherapy followed by concurrent chemoradiotherapy in stage N2-3 nasopharyngeal carcinoma: Phase 3 multicentre randomised controlled trial. BMJ 2025 Apr 15; 389:e081557. (https://doi.org/10.1136/bmj-2024-081557)

141. Foss FM et al. Efficacy and safety of denileukin diftitox-cxdl, an improved purity formulation of denileukin diftitox, in patients with relapsed or refractory cutaneous T-cell lymphoma. J Clin Oncol 2025 Apr; 43:1198. (https://doi.org/10.1200/JCO-24-01549)

142. Haddad R et al. Atezolizumab in high-risk locally advanced squamous cell carcinoma of the head and neck: A randomized clinical trial. JAMA 2025 Mar 13; [e-pub]. (https://doi.org/10.1001/jama.2025.1483)

143. Liang Y-L et al. Adjuvant PD-1 blockade with camrelizumab for nasopharyngeal carcinoma: The DIPPER randomized clinical trial. JAMA 2025 Mar 13; [e-pub]. (https://doi.org/10.1001/jama.2025.1132)

144. Thariat J et al. Survival without quality of life deterioration in the GORTEC 2014-04 "OMET" randomized phase 2 trial in patients with head and neck cancer with oligometastases using stereotactic ablative radiation therapy (SABR) alone or chemotherapy and SABR. Int J Radiat Oncol Biol Phys 2025 Apr 1; 121:1194. (https://doi.org/10.1016/j.ijrobp.2024.11.084)

145. Cooperberg MR et al. When is prostate cancer really cancer? Freeof the National Cancer Institute, Volume 117, Issue 3, 402–405, https://doi.org/10.1093/jnci/djae200

146. André T et al. Nivolumab plus ipilimumab versus nivolumab in microsatellite instability-high metastatic colorectal cancer (CheckMate 8HW): A randomised, open-label, phase 3 trial. Lancet 2025 Feb 1; 405:383. (https://doi.org/10.1016/S0140-6736(24)02848-4)

147. Schram AM et al. Efficacy of zenocutuzumab in NRG1 fusion–positive cancer. N Engl J Med 2025 Feb 6; 392:566. (https://doi.org/10.1056/NEJMoa2405008)

148. Bu, F et a. Risk of Thyroid Tumors With GLP-1 Receptor Agonists: A Retrospective Cohort Study. Diabetes Care 2025;48(8):1386–1394. https://doi.org/10.2337/dc25-0154

149 Harborg S, et al. Postdiagnosis statin use and breast cancer mortality. JAMA Netw Open 2025 Oct 1; 8:e2538737. DOI: 10.1001/jamanetworkopen.2025.38737.

150. Campone, M et al. Vepdegestrant, a PROTAC Estrogen Receptor Degrader, in Advanced Breast Cancer. N Engl J Med 2025;393:556-568. DOI: 10.1056/NEJMoa2505725

151. Guarneri V, Lenihan DJ, Valero V, Durand JB, Broglio K, Hess KR, Michaud LB, Gonzalez-Angulo AM, Hortobagyi GN, Esteva FJ. Long-term cardiac tolerability of trastuzumab in metastatic breast cancer: the M.D. Anderson Cancer Center experience. J Clin Oncol. 2006 Sep 1;24(25):4107-15. doi: 10.1200/JCO.2005.04.9551. Epub 2006 Aug 14. Erratum in: J Clin Oncol. 2008 May 10;26(14): 2421. PMID: 16908934.

152. Butare A, Sutton T, Kantzler E, Kennedy KN, Tumin D, Honaker MD. Adjuvant Chemotherapy for High-Risk Stage II Colon Cancer: A Population-Based Study. J Gastrointest Cancer. 2025 Feb 13;56(1):63. doi: 10.1007/s12029-025-01186-z. PMID: 39945928; PMCID: PMC11825529.

153. Testa U, Sica S, Pelosi E, Castelli G, Leone G. CAR-T Cell Therapy in B-Cell Acute Lymphoblastic Leukemia. Mediterr J Hematol Infect Dis. 2024 Jan 1;16(1):e2024010. doi: 10.4084/MJHID.2024.010. PMID: 38223477; PMCID: PMC10786140.

154. Lötscher J, et al. Respiratory syncytial virus vaccination in adult allogeneic hematopoietic cell transplant recipients. JAMA 2025 Oct 2; [e-pub] 10.1001/jama.2025.16744.41037295

42. ABBREVIATIONS USED

ADT, androgen-deprivation therapy

AKT, Ak strain transforming

APL, acute promyelocytic leukemia

ARPI, androgen-receptor pathway inhibitors

ATRA, All-trans retinoic acid

BRAF, B-rapidly accelerated fibrosarcoma

BTK, Bruton's tyrosine kinase

CALR, calreticulin

CAR, chimeric antigen reactive

CDK, cyclin-dependent kinase inhibitor

CIPN, chemotherapy-induced peripheral neuropathy

CLL, chronic lymphocytic leukemia

CR, complete remission

CRC, colorectal cancer

CRIS, complete remission with incomplete hematologic recovery

CRS, cytokine release syndrome

CT, computed tomgraphy

CTTLN, CAR transgenic T-cell lymphoproliferative neoplasm

DH, double hit

DLBCL, diffuse large B cell lymphoma

ECOG, Eastern Co-operative Oncologt Group

EFS, event-free survival

ER, estrogen receptor

ESD, endoscopic submucosal dissection

FDA, (USA) Food and Drug administration

FLOT, fluorouracil, leucovorin, oxaliplatin, and docetaxel

FOL/FOX, folinic acid (leucovorin, FOL), fluorouracil (5-FU, F), and oxaliplatin (Eloxatin, OX)

FP, fluorinated pyrimidine

GC, gemcitabine and cisplatin

GEJ, gastroesophageal junction

HER2, human epidermal growth factor 2

HL, Hodgkin lymphoma

HR, hazard rate

HSCT, hematopoietic stem cell transplantation

HPV, human papilloma virus

ICANS, immune effector cell–associated neurotoxicity syndrome

ICI, Immune checkpoint inhibitor

IGVH, immunoglobulin heavy chain

JAK2, Janus kinase 2

LBCL, large B cell lymphoma

mCSPC, metastatic castration-sensitive prostate cancer

MET, mesenchymal–epithelial transition

MHC, major histocompatibility complex

MPL, myeloproliferative leukaemia

MRD, minimal residual disease

MRI, magnetic resonance imaging

MSI, microsatellite-instability

Nab, albumen-bound

NFkB, nuclear factor kappa-light chain-enhancer of activated B cells

NK, natural killer

NPC, nasopharyngeal carcinoma

OS, overall survival

PARP, poly(ADP-ribose) polymerase

PD-L1, programmed death ligand 1

PE, pulmonary embolism

PET, positron emission tomography

PFS, progression-free survival

PIK3C, phosphatidylinositol-4,5-bisphosphate 3-kinase catalytic subunit alpha

Pola-R-CHP, polatuzumab, rituximab, cyclophosphamide, doxorubicin, and prednisone

PTOTAC, proteolysis-targeting chimera estrogen receptor degrader

PSA, prostate-specific antigen

R/R, relapsed/refractory

RAS, rat sarcoma virus

R-CHOP, rituximab, cyclophosphamide, doxorubicin, vincristine, and prednisone

SBRT, stereotactic body radiotherapy

SERDS, selective estrogen-receptor degraders

SLL, small lymphocytic lymphoma

SLNB, sentinel lymph node biopsy

SOC, standard of care

TAM, tumor-associated macrophages

T-DM1, trastuzumab emtansine

TCR, T cell receptor

TKI, tyrosine kinase inhibitor

TME, tumor microenvironment

TNBC, triple-negative breast cancer

TNM, tumor, node , metastasis

TP53, tumor suppressor gene 53

TTF, tumor treatment field

VTE, venous thromboembolism

Made in the USA
Coppell, TX
05 November 2026

11315640R00098